According to the Thyroid Foundation of Canada, approximately two hundred million people in the world suffer from some form of thyroid disease. As Dr. Maccaro points out in her book, "more than 12 percent of Americans will develop a thyroid condition" during their lifetime. One of the unique features of this book is that it is written from the author's firsthand account of and lifelong battle with thyroid disease. Surviving thyroid cancer provides Dr. Maccaro with a passionate and personal perspective on thyroid disease. Her narrative takes it out of the abstract and casts the challenge of fighting thyroid disease in realistic terms. Further, Dr. Maccaro's background and training in naturopathy, along with her knowledge and understanding of traditional and integrative medicine, gives the reader a professional and credible reporting on the nature of thyroid disease, its prevalence, and how it can be treated and prevented.

Dr. Maccaro has been a colleague of mine for nearly ten years. She has appeared on my nationally syndicated health talk show a number of times. She always shows up prepared not only to talk about the topic but to help listeners take charge of their health. Just as she has done on my shows and in all of her previous books and writings, Dr. Maccaro will help her readers take charge of their health and win the battle against thyroid disease.

—Michael Garko, PhD
Nationally Syndicated Host and Producer,
Let's Talk Nutrition

Dr. Janet Maccaro is such an inspiration for women everywhere. She brings to the table so much knowledge and experience to all of us who have suffered from thyroid problems. Janet gets the mind-body concept and is exceptional at giving women power over this silent epidemic. I love how relatable this book is and how it gives us our power back. Thank you, Janet! #powerisinyourcourt!

—Holly Lerma, DDS

I've known Dr. Janet for many years and continue to be blown away by her knowledge of everything related to natural health and body wellness, especially regarding thyroid disease. This book is a much-needed resource for all people, especially women, to not only understand the truth about thyroid disease, but also how to address it naturally and holistically. She is one of the rare people who actually brings all the factual evidence, knowledge, and PhD expertise necessary combined with the real-life experiences of walking through this issue herself. I cannot recommend my friend Dr. Janet highly enough. Her work, expertise, books, and especially this latest book is as good as it gets.

—Bob Dutko
Nationally Syndicated Radio Host,
The Bob Dutko Show
Crawford Broadcasting Company
WMUZ Radio—Detroit 103.5FM

DR. JANET'S GUIDE TO THYROID HEALTH

JANET MACCARO, PhD, CNC

SILOAM

Most Charisma House Book Group products are available at special quantity discounts for bulk purchase for sales promotions, premiums, fund-raising, and educational needs. For details, write Charisma House Book Group, 600 Rinehart Road, Lake Mary, Florida 32746, or telephone (407) 333-0600.

Dr. Janet's Guide to Thyroid Health
by Janet Maccaro, PhD, CNC
Published by Siloam
Charisma Media/Charisma House Book Group
600 Rinehart Road
Lake Mary, Florida 32746
www.charismahouse.com

Cover design by Vincent Pirozzi
Design Director: Justin Evans

Visit the author's website at www.DrJanetPhD.com.

Library of Congress Cataloging-in-Publication Data:
Names: Maccaro, Janet C.
Title: Dr. Janet's guide to thyroid health / Janet Maccaro.
Other titles: Guide to thyroid health
Description: First edition. | Lake Mary, Florida : Siloam, [2016] | Includes
bibliographical references.
Identifiers: LCCN 2015045978| ISBN 9781629986364 (trade paper) | ISBN
9781629986371 (e-book)
Subjects: LCSH: Thyroid gland--Diseases.
Classification: LCC RC655 .M2045 | DDC 616.4/4--dc23
LC record available at http://lccn.loc.gov/2015045978

While the author has made every effort to provide accurate Internet addresses at the time of publication, neither the publisher nor the author assumes any responsibility for errors or for changes that occur after publication.

16 17 18 19 20 — 9 8 7 6 5 4 3 2
Printed in the United States of America

Our bodies are wonderfully and fearfully made. When balance is lost, we begin to live more fearfully and less wonderfully.

I dedicate this work to all who are suffering from the "invisible illness" called thyroid disease. May this book lift the veil and show you why you feel the way you do, lead you to proper diagnosis, and help you achieve the goal of optimal treatment.

I have experienced life from the dulled and painful perspective of undiagnosed thyroid disease. I am writing this book from my heart to yours. If I can help you identify and treat this stealthy thief that robs you of energy, vitality, and so much more, then to God be all the glory.

CONTENTS

ACKNOWLEDGMENTS

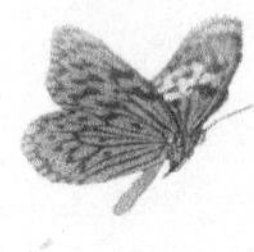

I WOULD LIKE TO acknowledge all the wonderful healthcare professionals who have arrived on the scene in the past few years. Many of these dedicated medical professionals have been faced with opposition from their peers as they seek to educate their patients as well as the general public on the devastating effect and the root causes of thyroid disease—particularly when it stems from autoimmunity: Amy Myers, MD; David Perlmutter, MD; Datis Kharrazian, DHSc, DC, MS; Josh Axe, DNM, DC, CNS; "Health Detective" Chris Kresser, MS, LAc; and Mary J. Shomon. These dedicated souls have dealt with thyroid issues or autoimmunity issues personally or by watching a family member struggle, as I have. I am very grateful that they all have arrived and collectively are changing the way thyroid disease is viewed and treated. I am also grateful for the very informative websites Hypothyroidmom.com and StopTheThyroidMadness.com, which have made great inroads when it comes to enlightening and alerting people of the importance of finding this disease sooner rather than later. Thyroid disease is a complicated issue, and it takes an army to conquer the myriad of factors that contribute to the unwellness it brings to a person's life. I am honored to be a part of this ever-growing army, and I salute my colleagues. I wear my "battle scar" with pride!

FOREWORD

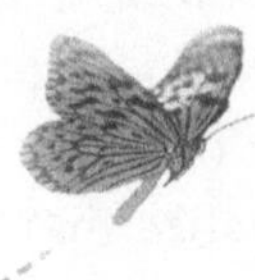

THERE IS NOTHING as frustrating as constantly feeling sick, barely able to get through the day, functioning at a mere fraction of normal, knowing in your heart that something "bad" is wrong with you...and having doctor after doctor fail to establish a diagnosis.

One of the most undiagnosed, misdiagnosed, and mistreated conditions is thyroid disease, and it is this giant that Dr. Janet Maccaro has chosen to attack. I have a confession...when I was sent this book, I planned on only scanning it. After all, I've been a practicing physician for more than forty years, and I've dealt with my share of patients with thyroid disease, so I assumed that the material would already be familiar to me. Well, I couldn't have been more wrong!

First of all, I was almost immediately captivated when I realized that every word of this story was based on her personal experience, as well as the personal experience of her children, with the horrors of thyroid disease *and* the myriad of complications of the conditions. The realization that she and her family had actually lived with these problems every hour of every day was so compelling that I read every word of the book.

Dr. Maccaro obviously researched the entire subject of thyroid disease while seeking answers through mainstream medicine and alternative medical channels. Her ability to document the symptoms and describe the complex interrelationships of the thyroid hormone and its effects on all of the other organ systems is amazing, especially when you realize that this book is written in a form that the average person without any medical training can understand.

The bottom line is that *everyone* should read this book, as this condition can affect you, your family, and your friends without anyone diagnosing it accurately. In this day and age, we all have to be part of the process of medical care. This book can give you the information to recognize many of the more subtle symptoms and possibly save years of anguish before the diagnosis is made.

Kudos to Dr. Maccaro for this incredible true story!

Respectfully submitted,

—DENNIS H. HARRIS, MD

Preface

THAT "BUTTERFLY" IN YOUR NECK

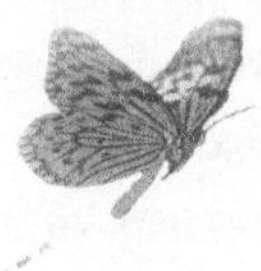

A BUTTERFLY IS A beautiful thing to behold. It symbolizes breaking free from a cocoon and emerging transformed and changed forever.

There is also a "butterfly" in your neck that helps your entire body perform beautifully—until something somewhere in your system goes haywire, changing your life forever.

Thyroid illnesses, such as hypothyroidism, autoimmune thyroid problems, and thyroid cancer, are increasing at epidemic rates. I believe thyroid problems are the most underdiagnosed conditions in our modern world. Unfortunately many conventional physicians are not educated on the physiology of the thyroid gland and fail to order the appropriate tests to evaluate thyroid function.

You are about to learn there is more to evaluating a thyroid gland than simply measuring TSH levels. This information will possibly save you from decades of illness that eludes the most skilled practitioners as its symptoms can have you referred to one specialty doctor after another. When your thyroid is not working properly, there is a ripple effect that touches each and every organ system and cell in your body. If you are suffering from hypothyroidism, your life is spent in a cocoon of brain fog, body aches, cold extremities, dry skin, constipation, anxiety, depression, and weight gain.

Hypothyroidism, when not optimally addressed, can be a major contributor to many of today's most common degenerative diseases, including heart disease, obesity, autoimmune disorders, and cancer. With thyroid disease your daily prayer consists of asking for help to be able to emerge from your cocoon healthy, vibrant, and full of energy. You long to be able to spread your wings and fly!

I am about to teach you all that I have learned during my long struggle with undiagnosed thyroid disease that spread over decades and ultimately became thyroid cancer. It is ironic that it happened to someone who has written ten health books and has lived a very clean life. But this goes to show you this disease is no respecter of persons. It happens to people in all walks of life. Many are suffering in silence. Many have given up hope of living a normal life ever again. I want to help break you free from the cocoon of this invisible illness. My goal here is for my journey to serve as the wind beneath your beautiful wings, empowering you and enabling you to fly on to your God-given destiny in vibrant health!

Dr. Janet's Guide to Thyroid Health is the story of the journey I lived for more than forty years with undiagnosed Hashimoto's thyroid disease, which ended with the loss of my thyroid due to cancer. My two daughters have also dealt with thyroid disease and its devastating effects on their lives. My youngest had to surrender her thyroid gland to a surgeon's scalpel due to thyroid cancer as well. You can understand why I want to offer this complete guide to the masses. I am completely dedicated to sharing with you all I have learned. No trial is ever wasted!

YOU AND YOUR UNDIAGNOSED THYROID DISEASE

THYROID DISEASE IS an often undetected, underdiagnosed, and undertreated disease that leaves countless sufferers unhappy and unhealthy. It is not unusual to go decades without being diagnosed or optimally treated. Living with thyroid disease can be very bewildering. Consider the following questions in light of your own experience:

- Do you have increased susceptibility to colds and other viral infections plus difficulty recovering from them?
- Does your hair fall out easily?
- Do you have dry skin or brittle, dry hair?
- Do you have low body temperature?
- Have you lost the outer third of your eyebrows?
- Do you heal slowly from wounds?
- Do you have cold hands and feet?
- Are you constipated?
- Are you depressed?
- Are you anxious or suffering from panic attacks?

- Are you gaining weight, no matter what you do to lose it?

If you answered yes to many of these questions, you could be facing thyroid disease.

THE DOWNWARD SPIRAL

Thyroid disease is an insidious affliction, and one of its hallmark symptoms is slowing down. This slowing can be felt from your head to your toes. Your reflexes slow down (when I was a child, my doctors always remarked, "You must not be alive," because I had no reflexes), and even adjusting to the environment becomes difficult.

Hypothyroid people often carry sweaters with them. Growing up in Florida, I loved to bask in the sun for hours, but never once did I sweat. I had no problem wearing a coat or sweater in the spring, even after I made the move to Arizona in 2006. The weather was hot, hot, hot to most people, but to me it was not, not, not! I know now it was because my metabolic rate was slow.

When your thyroid slows you down, it affects your digestive system. Constipation, bloating, and poor appetite can be a daily battle to overcome. Many women I have helped over the years have said they only have one or two bowel movements a week. (Yes, you read that right!) This is a clear sign you need to have your thyroid function checked.

Weight gain is always associated with the slowing-down process. A weight gain of ten to fifteen pounds in the period of one year even though you are not eating any differently is typical of a thyroid connection. I gained twenty-five pounds that I could not shake.

The most profound symptom of thyroid disease that I felt and that most people report is fatigue. It is not simply being tired. Rather, it is a deep-down feeling of lethargy, sluggishness, and dullness. I found that just moving around felt different. It took more effort just to move.

People with hypothyroidism often have high cholesterol. My cholesterol was 357 when I was only twenty-one years old. It remained high for decades. Not once did a physician consider it could be my thyroid acting up (or should I say, *not* acting up). If your cholesterol has been high for most of your life, have yourself checked for hypothyroidism or autoimmune thyroid issues. Why resort to taking a statin medication that has side effects when the root cause could be a faltering thyroid gland?

Muscle cramping and aching are also part of the hypothyroid journey. I can remember jumping up in the night with severe cramping in my feet. It was very painful, to say the least. Many people visit massage therapists and chiropractors in an attempt to make the discomfort end. I was one of them. Unfortunately it will never end unless you are optimally treated.

You may also find yourself dropping things, feeling uncoordinated or klutzy. This is yet another manifestation of hypothyroidism. This "dropsy" symptom is caused by hypothyroidism's effect on your brain, namely your cerebellum.[1]

I once had a skin-care specialist tell me she had never seen anyone with skin as dry as mine. With thyroid issues your skin can feel dry and coarse. The heels of your feet, your elbows, and even your knees can crack from the lack of moisture in your skin. You may notice puffiness around your eyes and that your face has taken on a rounder appearance. Even your tongue may swell and enlarge. This can happen if you have myxedema, which is a thickening of your tissues and skin.

"Is that you?" Many people asked me that question when I

called them on the phone, because my voice changed as my thyroid disease progressed. This was because Hashimoto's disease and the inflammation it caused to my thyroid gland affected my vocal cords and made me sound a little hoarse at times. If you have a large nodule or goiter, your voice can have a raspy or husky quality also.

My hair has always been coarse and dry, but I attributed it to having naturally curly hair. I remember one instance when I was a teenager and a boy I was dating said to me, "You have really dry hair. Why don't you use a conditioner?" The truth was I spent hours on my hair, trying to make it shiny and smooth! But when you have thyroid issues, your hair can become dry, brittle, thin, and less shiny. Some women even lose a lot of hair and are alarmed to see handfuls of it on the shower floor or in their hairbrush.

You may notice you do not have to shave your legs as often. (That was great for me, because being Italian means being a professional leg shaver!) You may lose the outer third of your eyebrows, and that is no fun, though the upside is that an astute physician can recognize this symptom quickly and have your thyroid levels checked.

"Where did I put that?" You may find yourself asking that question daily. This is because hypothyroidism can make you feel out of it or spacey. You may find your concentration is not what it used to be and that you have to read something over and over to comprehend it. Thankfully this will improve, as will all of the symptoms I mentioned, with optimal thyroid treatment.

Mirror, Mirror, on the Wall

Take a look at yourself in the mirror. Has your face changed since you have not been feeling like your old self? Find an old photo (but not too old) and pay attention to any of the following changes that may indicate an underfunctioning thyroid:

- Face: puffy, full, skin pads around the eyelids
- Hair: dull, limp, dry
- Complexion: pale, yellowish, or porcelainlike
- Lips: swollen, more purple, tongue may be enlarged
- Eyebrows: outer third missing
- Expression: dull, sad, depressed
- Skin: dry, thick, peeling, cracked elbows and heels

This is truly a case when you can be your own doctor—and many times you must be when it comes to getting your diagnosis. The mirror does not lie, and you know your body better than anyone else. After all it is your flesh suit and earthly home. You know when something is amiss. When it comes to getting a proper diagnosis, you have to do what I refer to as PUSH—*Push Until Something Happens!*

It's Time to Act

Does any of this sound like you? If so, you're not alone. If you have these symptoms—and trust me, there are many more—but your doctor has told you that you're just fine, you could be one of the millions of undiagnosed sufferers of the "silent epidemic" called thyroid disease.

One in eight women will develop thyroid disease.[2] Chances are that if you feel unwell most of the time and the cause has not been found, the butterfly-shaped gland in your neck is fluttering too slow or too fast or is under attack by your immune system.

You know your body. And you are the one who must not take no for an answer when you know something is wrong. This book will arm you with the education you need to push until something happens, so you and your health-care provider can get to a proper diagnosis. Your life depends on it. Consider these statistics:

- Various sources now report anywhere from twenty million to as many as sixty million Americans, most of them women, have some form of thyroid disease.[3]
- More than 12 percent of Americans will develop a thyroid condition.[4]
- Women are five to eight times more likely than men to have thyroid problems.[5]
- Up to 60 percent of those with thyroid disease are unaware of their condition.[6]
- Cases of thyroid cancer are on the rise, with papillary cancer making up 70 to 80 percent of the cases.[7]

Undiagnosed thyroid disease can ruin your quality of life and put you at risk for serious conditions such as cardiovascular disease, osteoporosis, infertility, and more. Although the thyroid gland is relatively small, the hormone it produces influences every cell, tissue, and organ in your body.

Thyroid dysfunction robs you of life. I know this all too well. I will share with you in the next chapter how my two daughters and I each suffered the devastating effects of undiagnosed autoimmune thyroid disease. To make matters worse, my youngest daughter and I were both diagnosed with thyroid cancer after being dismissed by more than twenty physicians in three states. Two of them said it was impossible to have autoimmune thyroid disease and thyroid cancer at the same time. Sadly they were wrong.

I pushed more than twenty doctors for years until my daughters and I were diagnosed. My youngest daughter had progressed to stage 3 papillary thyroid cancer when she was finally diagnosed. This is not acceptable. It should not have taken decades to find the cause! Both conventional and alternative medicine failed to diagnose us for years. I even went to two of the most respected clinics in the world and they missed it.

My goal here is to not let this happen to you and your loved ones. My prayer is that you do not have to endure years of vague and dismissed symptoms that chip away at the quality of your life. It has been said that only those who have experienced it can teach it. I am here to teach it! My mission is to bring you my years of research along with my personal experience to help you recognize thyroid disease early, potentially saving you decades of misery, loss of vibrant health, and your life.

I am not trying to challenge the pharmaceutical industry or the medical profession. My goal is to empower you, educate you, and help you become proactive in terms of finding this elusive disease. The advice I give to you in this book is based upon my long and arduous journey to find the root cause and diagnosis of autoimmune thyroid disease in my children and myself. The information I share with you is not meant for "peer review" but rather to serve as a guide to help you dialogue with your health-care provider so you can obtain optimal thyroid health sooner rather than decades later.

Your life is waiting. Let's help you get it back.

Chapter 1

MY STORY

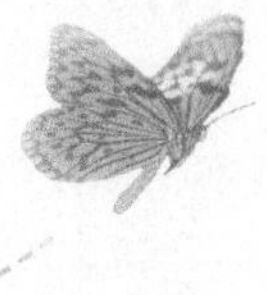

AS WITH MY previous books, I would like to give you an account of why and how this book came to be. You will find that it is bittersweet. I endured much illness throughout my life. The good news is that it all ultimately led me to my profession as a natural health author and educator. I have always been able to help others, and I feel that it is my true calling. I love to find the root cause of illness, and I enjoy spending hours in research in order to help others. This has been my passion for my entire life. I have always believed in the saying, "Follow your passion, and it will take care of you."

The good news is that it did. And now it is my commission to help take care of you.

My Rock Bottom

In 2007, after spending much time and energy writing, speaking, promoting my books, appearing on radio and television shows, and taking care of my family, I crashed. Hit a wall. Fell off a cliff. I could not function at all. I was in trouble.

Here's a little bit of my history. I was born prematurely. I was not breast-fed—something I've since learned is more important than I ever realized—and I had problems keeping food down. I was very sickly as a young girl. I had frequent strep throat infections that led to rheumatic fever, measles,

German measles, Epstein-Barr virus, and even diphtheria! I lived on antibiotics. I was very frail and skinny.

My body temp was 96.7 degrees for most of my life. Normally our body temperature is 98.6. That means my parents and my doctor did not realize how sick I was when I would have a fever of 100 degrees. The truth was, it was much higher than it seemed, and I was very sick.

I always loved warm blankets, sweaters, and coats, and was probably considered strange when I wore them way too early in the fall and packed them away way too late in the spring. I was always cold. Growing up in Daytona Beach, Florida, I spent hours sunning myself at the beach because it made me feel good. I used to tell my mother that I was "charging my battery" when she told me I spent too much time in the sun. Little did I know I was truly helping my body, not just getting an awesome tan.

As a teenager severe anxiety started just before my cycle each month. It manifested as shortness of breath and feeling hyper. I developed candida infections all over my body from all of the antibiotics I had to take. I craved sugar and carbs, but then I felt drowsy. I was fatigued and started to gain weight. My doctor said it was stress due to my parents' divorce. No one looked further. No one looked deeper. That cost me many years and my quality of life.

When I married at age twenty, I felt unwell as I walked down that aisle. Was it nerves again? This was a feeling of unwellness I would learn to live with as the years passed and as I raised my three children. I lived with fatigue, anxiety, cold feet and hands, constipation, dizziness, a slow heart rate, brain fog, strange sensations all over my body, an inability to sweat, shortness of breath, and many more symptoms as I tried to care for my family. I pushed myself, overcompensating for what I felt happening inside. I forced myself to be superwoman, when all the time I was not well and no doctor could tell me why.

I tried many things to feel better. I exercised whenever possible and took herbs, vitamins, and minerals, which helped for a time. But as the decades passed, this feeling of unwellness intensified as life issues became overwhelming and hormones declined. In other words, as I grew older and the things in life that shake you to your core happened, I broke down physically. After raising my family, going to school, writing ten books in ten years, lecturing, and giving my all to help others heal their bodies, minds, and spirits, I was broken and did not know if I could be fixed. I tried to outrun this feeling of unwellness that had haunted me since my early teen years. It had a hold on me, and it clearly wasn't going to let go.

An Unrelenting Search

It was then that I made a huge change in my life in order to save it. I moved to Arizona from Florida. I felt that I had to go to the desert, and thus began what I call my "wilderness experience." I consulted with the top doctors in Arizona for five solid years, and not one knew what to do for me. At the same time my youngest daughter, who became unwell in her teen years also, moved to Arizona with me so we could find help together.

I spent hours upon hours researching symptoms, diseases, syndromes, and specialists, all while suffering from one infection after another and from depression, anxiety, body pain, and unbelievable fatigue. But all my blood work was normal, they said, with just a few inflammatory markers. My daughters' tests looked much like mine.

How could we be so sick if the blood work was OK?

Their answer was stress. Over and over all we heard was,

"Oh, you're female. You moved across country, and you're just stressed out."

"Go for a walk. Exercise. Meet people," they said.

Then one night during my research I came across an autoimmune thyroid disease called Hashimoto's thyroiditis. The symptoms matched mine and those of my girls, and I found that most doctors do not routinely check for it.

I grabbed all my lab reports and noticed that the special tests they do for Hashimoto's were never done for me. Over and over again only the thyroid-stimulating hormone (TSH) was tested, never any antibodies to determine if autoimmune thyroiditis was the culprit in the destruction of our health and life.

Why?

It was interesting to note that Hashimoto's thyroiditis tends to be hereditary. That fact really crystallized when my oldest daughter in Florida became ill at the same time. Now all three of us were ill, and no concrete answers were forthcoming.

It has been said that a mother is only as happy as her saddest child. Well, let me tell you, we were all pretty sad. Thousands of dollars and hundreds of hours were spent trying to catch this thief that was robbing me and my girls of our health and quality of life.

Desperate for help I went to an urgent-care doctor and asked for help. The doctor ran a thyroid panel, complete with thyroid peroxidase antibody (TPO) and thyroglobulin antibody (TgAb) autoimmune markers. Three days later I was diagnosed with Hashimoto's thyroiditis, an autoimmune thyroid disease that had plagued me for four decades.

That was step one in my story. The enemy was found.

But I knew by my research that Hashimoto's disease tends to be hereditary, so I made sure both of my daughters were also tested. Their tests came back with thyroid antibodies, meaning my two girls shared my diagnosis. Of course I was not thrilled about this, but I was relieved that the enemy that was seeking to destroy us had been unmasked.

We were now among the millions of women who deal with this insidious and often misunderstood illness, as evidenced by the literal parade of doctors who waved us by when we presented them with a myriad of chronic issues such as frequent bladder and sinus infections, foggy thinking, headaches, insomnia, and panic attacks—to name just a few of the more than two hundred possible symptoms.

I was relieved this "stealthy robber" of our health was finally found. What I didn't realize was that this was only the beginning of yet another season of battle.

Another Long Road

Once a diagnosis was made, we sought the help of several endocrinologists whose treatment recommendations were as different as their office decor. It was a bewildering experience. The advice ranged from "You don't need treatment since your TSH is in range" to "Let's put you on Synthroid, and you will be as good as new." Alternative doctors suggested we take desiccated thyroid hormone medication, such as Armour, Nature-Throid, Westhroid, and WP Thyroid, since they are most like the thyroid hormones we make ourselves. (You will learn more about these later.)

You need to know that over the years I tried everything I knew to help my daughters and myself. They depended on me to help them. I had to sort this out for the three of us—and ultimately for you, my readers, too. I had no idea what was about to unfold in our lives. I wish I would have fastened my seat belt tighter, because our ride was wild, stressful, and expensive, requiring me to rely more heavily on my faith than at any other time in my life. My babies were sick, and I was functioning with one hand tied behind my back.

Months passed as we tried one therapy after another. Each health professional was sure that his or her recommendation was the correct one. Unfortunately something very important was missing.

I wish I had known then, when my girls and I were going through it, what I am going to teach you now. It would have spared us so much agony. But I trust that everything happens for a reason and a season, and that every test has a testimony. Writing this book seven years later is proof positive.

Since my daughters and I were not springing back to health as many of the doctors promised we would, I knew I had to dig deep. I had to be a better doctor than the doctors I was seeing. I had to become more educated on the causes of autoimmunity than I had been in previous years.

As I researched, I found that inflammation plays a huge role in the autoimmune picture. I also learned that autoimmunity begins in the gut. What causes that inflammation? Many things: antibiotics, NSAIDS, stress, steroid use, and gluten, to name some of the major factors.

Upon further research I also found that Hashimoto's thyroiditis has a very strong connection to gluten sensitivity. In fact many people with Hashimoto's disease also have another autoimmune condition called celiac disease. Celiac patients cannot have gluten at all or they can suffer extreme brain and body symptoms.

The deeper I dug, the more I realized that even though we all were on thyroid medication, that was not going to be enough, because we still felt unwell. Eventually my research would back up what I was feeling.

It turns out that Hashimoto's is really not a thyroid disease, as I had pictured it in my mind previously, but rather an autoimmune disease. This fact made our diagnosis much more frightening at the time. Our immune system, the very army that is designed to fight foreign invaders such as bacteria, viral assaults, cancer, and more, was now turning against all three of us. Its mission? Destroy the thyroid gland and, along with it, other tissues and organ systems in the body. Autoimmune disease is a systemic disease. Once you have one, the stage is set for more.

What was our particular trigger? How did all three of us become ill at the same time? (Or did we?) Yes, we all were ill, but we each had vague symptoms for years before we really crashed.

Every time I researched causes for autoimmune disease, stress came up as a huge trigger, precipitating cases of lupus, rheumatoid arthritis, Hashimoto's thyroiditis, Graves' disease, vitiligo, alopecia, and more.

It made sense. All three of us had tons of stress for different reasons during the years leading up to our health crisis. As time went on, our ability to cope diminished daily. I had always chalked my reaction up to stress to my being a high-strung Italian.

Oh, and speaking of being Italian, for years I cooked pasta in any configuration you can think of—lasagna, manicotti, baked ziti, and more. Oh, and the bread—warm Italian bread was always a must. There was a *lot* of gluten going on!

I marked genetics as trigger number one, followed by stress, and it looked like my next piece of this agonizing puzzle was to get a test for gluten allergy. Wouldn't you know it, my youngest daughter and I were found to have high gliadin antibodies in our blood and in our stool. (She was a real trooper when I demanded she do the stool test—it's not very fun.) The recommendation by the labs was to eliminate gluten for the rest of our lives.

Continuing on, I learned that wheat gluten can cause severe inflammation in the gut, leading to what's known as "leaky gut." Once you have leaky gut, proteins, sugars, and starches from the foods you eat can enter your bloodstream and set off an alarm telling your immune system to attack these invaders, only it's a false alarm. Instead of real invaders, your immune system attacks the foods you eat that are simply leaking out of your inflamed gut, which has become riddled with open cell junctions.

Now picture this happening twenty-four hours a day—eating gluten such as breads, pasta, and cakes, which inflames your gut, which causes leaky gut and over time causes your immune system's army to be pushed too far, resulting in mutiny on the body in an all-out attack on you.

At that point I had three very important pieces of the puzzle figured out. I was sure I was on my way to having all three of us up and running, but it would take time.

THE DREADED "C" WORD

Then I read about thyroid nodules and how common they are, especially in Hashimoto's disease. They often happen in straightforward cases of hypothyroidism as well. I felt that we should have scans performed to get a baseline and to find out what was indeed going on with the "butterflies" in our necks.

I went first. The result was a single, solitary nodule. It looked OK. They said, "Let's watch it." I agreed. I was more concerned about having my daughter's thyroid scanned than my own.

You will learn more about this later, but I will tell you now that her scan was not good. Just by ultrasound alone and before a biopsy, I was told there was a strong possibility she had thyroid cancer and that it looked aggressive, given her age. Keep in mind that we were told by several other doctors at that time that we were just stressed—that we needed to make friends, get massages, dry-brush our bodies, have vitamin C treatments, and take saunas; one doctor had me drink a nice big glass of water infused with ozone and then gave me an ozone IV. There were several other outrageous treatment plans that drained my bank account and my mind. I always pulled myself back to sound reasoning at the end of each day. Thank God, because if I'd listened to all of them, it may have been too late for my girl!

We had to act fast. Her surgery was performed right away. The outcome? Stage 3 papillary thyroid cancer. She then had to undergo radioactive iodine therapy (RAI), which involves swallowing a radioactive iodine capsule in order to kill off any remaining thyroid tissue and cancer cells that were missed during her surgery. She was in isolation at home for several days, as she was radioactive. Everything she used, touched, or wore had to be bagged and disposed of in a special way.

It was heartbreaking to watch her go through this after being so ill for so many years from the autoimmune part of this disease. I thought we had found the answer: eliminate the triggers and autoimmunity would reverse. But cancer? She had to get rid of this beast first before I could help her implement any of the other necessary lifestyle and dietary changes.

The surgeon assured us that once she got that thyroid out, my daughter would feel much better. Unfortunately she felt worse. The surgery caused her to lose her voice for several weeks, and the body scan after her RAI treatment caused her organs to feel as if they were heating up. She was given a few different kinds of thyroid medications ranging from the synthetic, such as Synthroid, to the more bioidentical, such as Armour and Nature-Throid. She was told she needed to be patient and that this adjustment would take time.

While she was waiting for her medication to do something, I decided it was time for me to investigate my thyroid nodule more thoroughly. I had another ultrasound performed, and this time a new radiologist detected a worrisome feature: microcalcifications, which are tiny bits of calcium found often in malignancy, particularly in papillary thyroid cancer. He also noticed my nodule had grown ever so slightly, from four millimeters to seven millimeters.

I told him my daughter had just been diagnosed with an aggressive stage 3 papillary cancer, and asked him for a fine-needle biopsy. He agreed but told me he probably could not get a good sample since the nodule was under one centimeter in diameter. He also told me I was probably fine since it had not changed much and was very small. I pushed, though, because the research I did previously told me a solitary nodule with microcalcifications is very likely to be malignant.

The radiologist knew me well by this time due to my tenacity concerning getting my daughter diagnosed. He knew I was going to push him hard, so he agreed. He very skillfully biopsied my seven-millimeter nodule in five different areas, and he told me not to worry. After all, what were the chances of my having thyroid cancer at the same time as my daughter? I went home very unsettled and waited for his call.

The next day the phone rang. I knew what was coming. Let me tell you, even if you suspect that you have it, no one is ever prepared to hear those three words: "You have cancer." In this case I heard, "You have cancer *too*."

The doctor told me to find a surgeon and get it taken care

of as soon as possible. I was stunned, to say the least. I actually sat down and pinched myself very hard to make sure this was not some crazy, stress-induced parallel universe where the things you would never want to happen do happen.

So here we were, my daughter struggling to recover from her surgery and trying to get thyroid hormones to replace what her diseased thyroid used to make, while I was facing thyroid cancer surgery at the same time. I am the mothership. I did not have time for this!

I had the surgery and was found to have stage 1 papillary thyroid cancer. My youngest daughter and I had to face new challenges together as we joined the ranks of people who live without a thyroid gland.

A Multilayered Recovery

Both of my daughters depended on me to help them figure out this health crisis. I was really hard on myself during this time. I blamed myself for not pushing harder or sooner, for not researching more or finding more doctors. I questioned my chosen career as a natural health educator and consultant. I questioned everything except my faith in God.

The season of recovery was very hard because the endocrinologists we visited were very conventional and had only one plan for thyroid disease: a choice between two synthetic thyroid medications. We were not doing well, and these doctors had no answers. Again the "stress card" came up.

I researched everything I could on the thyroid and often knew more than our doctors. This wasn't working well for us, believe me. No doctor likes to be questioned, even if you do it kindly and with a smile. I insisted on answers, and they didn't have them.

In books I have written in the past, I talk about the importance of adrenal gland health and how crucial the adrenals are in helping to keep us strong and healthy, especially during times of stress. There is also a strong connection between the adrenal glands and the health of the thyroid. If your thyroid is malfunctioning, your adrenals become taxed. If left unattended, this can ultimately lead to autoimmune disease, because the adrenal glands lose the ability to produce cortisol, which is essential for your body to be able to handle stress and keep inflammation under control.

As I went down the adrenal path more and more, I noticed that experts in the field often disagreed on thyroid treatment. It was either "Take a thyroid pill and don't worry about the adrenals," or "Work on the adrenals first and get them strong so the thyroid pill will be more effective." There was also the idea of working on both thyroid and adrenal health at the same time.

With all this conflicting information in my head and the stress of all this cancer talk, plus the surgeries, recoveries, medical bills, and not feeling any better, I had to find the way out of all of this, and soon. I went back to all my notes and went into prayer night after night. I researched unceasingly because our lives depended on it.

Most cases—90 percent—of adult thyroid disease cases are autoimmune, which means your immune system is attacking your thyroid.[1] If this applies to you, my goal here is to help you find out why. It can be overwhelming to face, but once each connecting factor is addressed—the triggers are acknowledged, the gut is healed, the diet is adjusted, and the thyroid and adrenals are supported—your life can turn around. Even though you may have lost your "butterfly," you still have your wings.

I am giving you this information so you can fly. Most of all, remember to push—for you, your daughters, your mother, your friends, and anyone you may see who is struggling. With this information, you may just help free them from the cocoon of chronic illness. My friend Mary pushed, and look what happened for her:

> It happened to me…
>
> At the age of fifty-seven I started feeling drained and sluggish. At the time I was working full time in retail. My doctor told me it was just age, but when I gained ten pounds for no apparent reason despite working out at least four days a week and watching what I ate, I began to doubt her theory.
>
> Months later, when I complained of my heart beating a little strangely, my doctor decided that I should see a cardiologist and be tested. The cardiologist found nothing wrong with my heart after performing an EKG and a stress test.
>
> My doctor then decided she would check for thyroid issues and also gave me a stern talk about my diet. My test came back showing that I had hypothyroidism, so she put me on Synthroid.
>
> I took it for about a year, when I noticed my hair was falling out rapidly and my legs were cramping all the time. In addition my heart was racing for no reason, and I just felt run down.
>
> About that time Dr. Janet and I reconnected. We had been friends for many years and had lost touch. I decided to call her and catch up. We got on the topic of my health. When I started telling her my health issues, not realizing she was having thyroid issues herself, she started asking me all sorts of questions and immediately suggested that I go back and tell my doctor that I needed further thyroid testing. Dr. Janet listed the blood tests that I needed to PUSH my doctor to order.

I waited for a while, thinking that my doctor would laugh at me for demanding these tests because, according to my doctor, all I needed to do was watch what I was eating and get more rest!

Four months later I was drying my hair one morning and a whole section fell out. I was now in panic mode! I called my doctor and told her I wanted to be seen that day! Her nurse listened to me, talked to the doctor, and the nurse called me right back. I told her what blood work I wanted done (the ones that Dr. Janet told me to get months before). Seeing how upset I was at the time, my doctor agreed to do the tests.

A week later my doctor called and told me that the blood work showed that I had Hashimoto's thyroiditis. The only thing she suggested that I do was to increase my medication. [She] offered no more help than that for me. She could tell me nothing about Hashimoto's.

I wonder how long or how sick would I have had to get before the correct blood work or more complete blood work was done. I am thankful that Dr. Janet and I connected again when we did. Dr. Janet has now instructed me to eliminate gluten for starters to help me on my wellness journey.

Chapter 2

GET TO KNOW YOUR THYROID

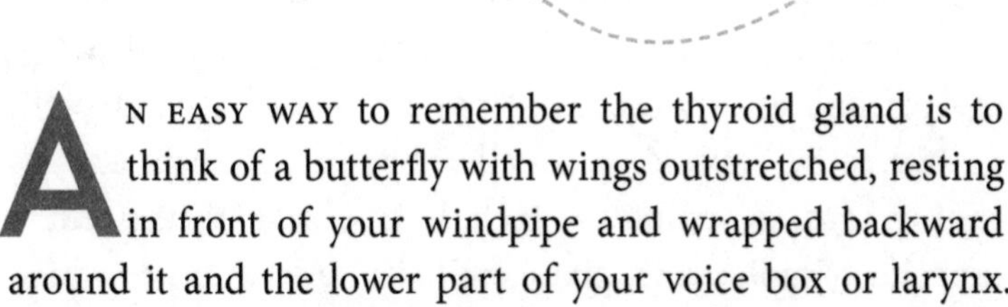

An easy way to remember the thyroid gland is to think of a butterfly with wings outstretched, resting in front of your windpipe and wrapped backward around it and the lower part of your voice box or larynx. When you swallow, your entire thyroid gland moves up and down with your Adam's apple.

My goal is to get you to know this butterfly very well, because your quality of life may depend on it. If your thyroid gland is not running optimally, neither are you! Let's educate you on just what your thyroid does and how it can find itself in peril.

What Is It?

It was the ancient Greeks who named the thyroid gland *thyreos*, which means "shield." This makes sense, since your thyroid's job is to protect or shield you from heat and cold by regulating your body temperature. This may seem like a simple way of looking at the thyroid, but the truth is that your thyroid just happens to be one of the most complex hormone-producing endocrine glands in your body. It is important that you understand how it functions in order to get well.

Your thyroid not only manages your body temperature but it has many other important jobs as well. The thyroid regulates your blood sugar, bone health, energy level, metabolism, menstrual cycle, cholesterol, heart rate, organ function, and stress hormone response.

HOW CAN IT GO WRONG?

The first thing to know concerning thyroid disorders is that they can manifest in two different patterns—an overactive thyroid and an underactive thyroid. When you deal with an overactive thyroid, it is called hyperthyroidism and its calling card of symptoms include trouble with concentration, heat intolerance, changes in bowels patterns (which includes frequent bowel movements), thinning skin, excessive sweating, increased appetite, unexpected weight loss even though you are still eating the same amount of food at each meal, nervousness, anxiety and restlessness, a visible lump in the throat (goiter), irregular menstrual periods, tremors, and rapid heartbeat.

Hypothyroidism, or an underactive thyroid, comes calling with equally uncomfortable symptoms such as loss of energy, hair loss, inappropriate weight gain despite exercise and healthy dietary practices, low body temperature with a feeling of always being cold, constipation, dry skin, heavy periods, and difficulty concentrating. The sad thing here is that many of these symptoms also are common in depressed persons, and therefore many people go for years not knowing that treating their underfunctioning thyroid gland or hypothyroidism could greatly improve the quality of their lives.

Please note that the majority of the information in this book addresses the underactive thyroid condition of hypothyroidism, primarily because that is the condition my daughters and I have faced, making it a primary focus of my many years of research. In addition, as you will soon see, hypothyroidism is linked to many other maladies, such as autoimmune diseases, gluten intolerance, leaky gut, and issues with the adrenal glands and blood sugar, and it has a great impact on other organs in the body. Each of these will be addressed in its own separate chapter later in the book.

What Are the Telltale Signs?

If you have undiagnosed thyroid disease, you will soon see a ripple effect that slowly erodes the quality of your life. Here are some of the signs it's happening to you.

"A slow in your go"

When your thyroid malfunctions, the amount of time it takes for food to move through your intestines increases. This causes constipation and thereby the potential for yeast overgrowth and gut infections that include harmful bacteria. The result is inflammation, leaky gut, and poor nutrient absorption. The stage is now set for food allergies and intolerance.

"Fat won't scat"

Low thyroid function makes it harder for your body to burn fat by shutting down the sites on your cells that metabolize fat. Even when your caloric intake is low and your time spent working out is high, you will have the inability to burn fat for energy due to the overall slowdown of your body's metabolism. If your thyroid malfunctions, your adrenal glands take a hit and cannot assist you with burning fat either, because they too have lost—or are in the process of losing—their "charge."

When your thyroid malfunctions, you make more fat than you burn. This raises your triglycerides, cholesterol, and LDL cholesterol. With low thyroid function, you have a hard time burning fat for fuel. In addition, your liver and gallbladder become sluggish, making it hard to metabolize fat and remove it from the body.

High cholesterol

Before I was diagnosed, I had a total cholesterol reading of 357 with very high triglycerides and an extremely high LDL level. Even though I weighed only 115 pounds when I was twenty years old, my body fat was a whopping 30 percent! The doctor said he must have measured wrong. Keep in mind that I was only twenty years old when I first received that high reading. My doctors back then said, "How odd. Well, you are young, so we won't worry about a heart attack."

I was able to lower my cholesterol levels with herbs and vitamins, but I was never able to get everything in a normal range. Now the answer is clear. Since my thyroid was under attack and unable to do its job in helping to clear fats from my body, my cholesterol was driven sky high.

My point here is that if you have high cholesterol, LDL levels, or triglycerides, get your thyroid checked and make sure to ask your health-care provider to check for autoimmune thyroid disease at the same time. This would mean asking for TPO and TgAb tests in addition to TSH.

Sluggish filtration

As I said, low thyroid function affects the way your liver and gallbladder work together to metabolize hormones, filter toxins, and clean your blood. When these by-products are sent to your gallbladder for final removal, low thyroid function impedes the process, which makes both the liver and gallbladder sluggish and congested, setting the stage for gallstones.

Here is an interesting side note: I once asked several clients who came to me because they were chronically ill and had their gallbladders removed if they had ever had their thyroid fully checked. Their answer was no. When they did, each had an underlying thyroid malfunction that was finally diagnosed.

Poor concentration

Thyroid disease can be likened to trying to think through oatmeal. An inability to concentrate, fuzzy thinking, poor memory, mood disorders, panic attacks, hypoglycemia, and lethargy all result from poor sugar metabolism and overtaxed adrenal glands.

Poor digestion

People with low stomach acid, heartburn, bloating, gas, and acid reflux should note that hypothyroidism and low stomach acid (commonly known as hydrochloric acid, or HCl) go hand in hand. Plenty of stomach acid is what you need to digest your food, to prevent food poisoning, and to get rid of nasty parasites and bad bugs. Contrary to what you may have thought, if you have sufficient stomach acid, you will not have heartburn. Heartburn comes from poorly digested food coming back up to say hello and painfully shooting up into your esophagus.

Your production of HCl depends on your production of a hormone called gastrin. Gastrin levels are typically low if you have low thyroid function. Without enough HCl, you will have poor absorption of B_{12}, magnesium, iron, and calcium, in addition to inflammation, infections, and painful lesions in the gastrointestinal tract. Adequate amounts of HCl will stimulate the gallbladder and pancreas to complete digestion and protect the environment and integrity of your entire gastrointestinal tract.

In the years before my Hashimoto's diagnosis I had an issue digesting proteins. As I researched, I found that one crucial job that a good supply of HCl does is help digest proteins. In people with thyroid malfunction a protein deficiency may occur because of this single and often overlooked causative factor. If you are downing antacids, have bloating, gas, reflux, or gallstones, or have even had your gallbladder removed, please have your thyroid checked now.

Iron deficiency

I remember an ad I used to see on television when I was a little girl that asked, "Do you have iron-poor blood?" Now I wonder if that problem could have been addressed through the thyroid gland rather than by taking the advertised tonic. When hypothyroidism leads to a deficiency in stomach acid, iron absorption is poor, leading to anemia. Anemia can also result from a B_{12} and folic acid deficiency, usually resulting from low stomach acid. In addition, low thyroid function is often connected to heavy menstrual periods. When you add this to poor iron absorption from low HCl, you have "iron-poor blood"—anemia caused by iron deficiency.

Case in point: my two daughters were both extremely anemic when they were finally diagnosed. They were told to take iron pills. Again, I am sharing vital information here. If you are anemic, have that thyroid checked, and while you are being treated, take a digestive enzyme with HCl with your meals.

High homocysteine

Hypothyroidism contributes to high homocysteine levels by compromising your liver's ability to manage it properly. Too much homocysteine, which is an amino acid, greatly increases your chances of a cardiac event or cardiovascular disease.

Viral infections

I want to stop and have you note here that my daughters and myself—all three of us—had subnormal body temperatures of 96.8 instead of 98.6. This is meaningful because your thyroid controls your body temperature.

Bacteria is very sensitive to temperature. If your body temperature is too low, you don't have enough body heat to keep harmful bacteria in check. When your thyroid is malfunctioning, your temperature will be too low to control the pathogenic insults waged upon your body each day. A consistently low temperature is a key indicator of thyroid problems and a major reason why thyroid sufferers have so many random infections and mystery sicknesses that seem unrelated.

To get to the bottom of this, I recommend that you take your temperature in the morning before rising. Then take it again later in the day. Chart your readings, as this will be yet another tool that helps you get to your correct diagnosis.

If my daughters and I had thyroids that were functioning correctly, we would have been spared having one infection after another, year after year. We all had friends that had very strong constitutions. They hardly ever came down with the common cold. Why did we struggle with all these bacterial and viral issues? Years later the answer would become clear: our thyroids were not up to the challenge of regulating our body temperatures, and our adrenal glands were being taxed, unbeknownst to us at the time.

With our thyroids fluttering to stay in the game; our adrenals sputtering to help handle our stress and quell inflammation; and yeast overgrowth weakening and inflaming our gut walls, causing them to leak like sieves, we each had a perfect storm that eventually led to autoimmune disease.

UPDATE

Why did three members of my family suffer from Hashimoto's thyroid disease, but only two of us went on to develop papillary thyroid cancer? There is emerging evidence that the culprit may not be as closely linked to genetics as originally thought, but instead related to a previous EBV (Epstein-Barr virus) infection. EBV has been found in the thyroid tissue of Hashimoto's and thyroid cancer patients.[1]

All three of us (my two daughters and I) had the virus in the 1980s. This virus is a tough one. It causes mono, but it also has been linked to lymphoma.

If you have Hashimoto's or any autoimmune disease, please ask for a blood test for EBV. Even if your results show a past EBV infection, the virus is still in your body, causing baffling symptoms that disrupt your life. Most physicians will not make this connection. If you are found to indeed have EBV, seek out a functional medicine doctor who will work with you to eradicate this virus or lessen the viral load. Conventional physicians may agree to prescribe a course of antiviral medication such as Acyclovir. To help overcome this virus, I recommend you read my book *90-Day Immune System Makeover.*

Chapter 3

YOU, YOUR DOCTOR, AND THE ELUSIVE BUTTERFLY

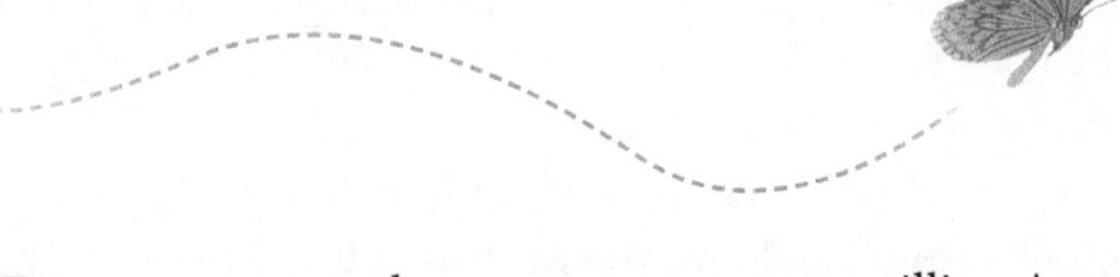

IT IS ESTIMATED that as many as twenty million Americans have a thyroid disease and more than half of them have no idea that they do.[1] My daughters and I were three of them. Thyroid disease is indiscriminate, striking the rich, the poor, the most average of us, and the most famous.

The good news is that today more and more people are getting diagnosed. However, there is still much work to do to raise awareness about thyroid disease and its many connections to other ailments we experience.

The hormones secreted by your thyroid affect each and every cell in your body, so it is not hard to figure out that the optimal functioning of your thyroid gland is crucial when it comes to maintaining the integrity and function of your entire body. When your thyroid health is compromised, even just a little, it often results in a plethora of symptoms and conditions that affect every organ in your body.

Consider this: How many people do you know who are always sick or have never been well? Do you know anyone who is a hypochondriac? With as many as two hundred symptoms affecting hypothyroid sufferers, you can see why their world is filled with health complaints and hypervigilance. How many beloved family members and friends that came before you went to their graves undiagnosed?

Looking back over my family tree's health histories, I

found out that both my aunts had high cholesterol and took medication for most of their lives. They were plagued with symptoms that mystified doctors for decades. They had all the symptoms of hypothyroidism and were never diagnosed or treated. From all that I know now, this means they suffered from adrenal involvement as well.

One of my aunts suffered with dizziness for forty years with no cause found. She was anemic, suffered from constipation, and had low body temperature. No physician looked at the thyroid-adrenal connection. That was in the 1960s and 1970s, before things came to light about the damage caused by untreated thyroid disease and how it can wreak havoc with every system in your body.

While I was going through the arduous journey with my daughters, I wondered if my aunts could have had Hashimoto's too. It was only after contacting my cousin that I found out she and her daughter were recently diagnosed with it. She told me she was feeling unwell many years before, but it took years for her to get diagnosed. So you can see there is a strong genetic link.

But genes do not have to express. If they do, stress is usually the trigger. Both my cousin and I underwent much stress in our personal lives before our diagnoses. Our adrenal glands were taxed, and the thyroid couldn't pitch in to keep up. And both of us had very high cholesterol, just as our aunts did.

A Confounding Diagnosis

Again, thankfully, thyroid disease is being spotted earlier in today's world. But unfortunately it can still take years to diagnose because the symptoms can be vague at first. What's more, thyroid disease, especially autoimmune thyroid disease, requires more than just a thyroid pill, and most health-care providers are unaware of this.

I cannot tell you how many times I was told, "Eat less and exercise more." I cannot tell you how insulted I felt when I heard this recommendation. After all, I was the author of almost a dozen health and nutrition books! When you are dealing with autoimmune thyroid disease, dietary and lifestyle generalities fly right out the window along with life as you once knew it. My diet was already good, but my ability to exercise was greatly hampered and then completely halted by this insidious affliction. It was hard for me to live with the mysterious symptoms and complaints I suffered from, let alone to raise my children, work, write, and take care of all the extracurricular activities that go along with family life. No matter how much effort I put into my diet and exercise routine, nothing changed. As a matter of fact, my symptoms only intensified. I felt as if my body was somehow betraying me.

If exercise, nutrition, and your doctor's advice can't seem to solve your problems, chances are very good that your thyroid is to blame. The additional secret you need to know here is this: low thyroid function is almost always secondary to some other condition, and most often it is adrenal stress. What's more, adrenal issues mean layers of underlying issues such as gut inflammation, blood sugar–handling issues, food intolerances, chronic bacterial or viral infections, hormonal imbalances, and environmental toxins.

You can see now why many people can go for years either undiagnosed, undertreated, or improperly managed. As I said in chapter 2, your thyroid function is very complex and affects your entire body; therefore, your entire body must be addressed if you are going to get well. The point for you to remember here is that your thyroid does not act alone, and when it goes down, it takes other body systems down with it!

Compounding this issue is the fact that these days, many doctors spend only a few minutes talking to patients, making it almost impossible to diagnose or sort out and unravel most cases of thyroid disease. Most doctors are content to throw a thyroid medication at an ailing thyroid, but this is no way to ensure getting to the root of the issue.

Additionally all three of us were told outrageous things by medical professionals, including a chief of endocrinology, as we pushed our way to diagnoses. Here are some of the most memorable:

- "You're just a closet eater, and you're in denial about it."
- "Are you doctor shopping?"
- "Maybe someone can help you—I can't."
- "You are just going to have to accept the fact that you are old now, and women get fat and frazzled when they age."
- "Do you have any friends?"
- "When is the last time you had sex?"
- "Why don't you take these symptoms to someone else?"
- "You're over fifty. Just relax and put yourself out to pasture. You have worked hard."
- "You just need a new purpose, that's all."
- "Maybe a psychic can help you."
- "Listen, we all get tired!"

- "Tired? You don't know what tired is. I work ninety hours a week."
- "I just got back from a seminar. I was the guest speaker. The problem with you is that you have a protozoan."
- "Your TSH says you're well, so accept it!"
- "You just want to be sick."
- "We'll recheck you in two years." (We had undiagnosed thyroid cancer then!)
- "Everyone's tired. Just have a cup of coffee and get going."
- "Isn't there a pill for that?"
- "Oh, a friend of mine has that same thing and she's fine."
- "Well, we'd all like to stay home and not work. Can I say I have that too?"
- "Your poor husband. That must be so hard on him."
- "If you had to get cancer, then thyroid cancer is the best one to get!" (Who knew I "had" to get cancer?)

Thankfully a new branch of medicine—called *functional medicine*—advocates a focus on finding the cause of the thyroid malfunction in the first place. This way of thought turned my life and health around. I have always been a staunch believer in alternative medicine, as evidenced by the many books I have previously written. But as it is said, "When the student is ready for more knowledge, the teacher appears." I now was ready to learn about functional medicine, a new field and train of thought that would help to save not only my life and my daughters' lives, but now yours as well.

Functional medicine differs greatly from conventional medicine. While prescription thyroid hormones can normalize your blood test results, they do not address the cause of your particular thyroid malfunction. Functional medicine seeks to find your cause. Now this is the way to practice medicine!

So consider: What is the cause of *your* thyroid condition? Here are some of the most common thyroid health destroyers:

- Hashimoto's thyroiditis (the most common cause of hypothyroidism in the United States)
- A gut infection
- Gluten sensitivity that has caused inflammation leading to autoimmunity
- Poor blood sugar control or insulin resistance
- Adrenal problems
- Hormonal imbalances
- Poor brain function
- Stealthy infections
- Unmanaged stress
- Food allergies
- Epstein-Barr virus

Finding your cause is the key to your recovery. It is interesting to note too that while one of these causes listed may be at the root of your thyroid woes, you need to work on *all* of the listed causes in order to recover your zest for life once again. It was all of these issues that plagued my daughters and me for years. Later on, after our diagnoses, the thyroid cancer surgeries, the recoveries, the thyroid hormone medication management, and hours upon hours of research, I learned that most people affected by thyroid disease, especially Hashimoto's, must address the body not with thyroid hormone medication alone but also with a concerted effort to address stress, diet (especially eliminating gluten), and gut health; look at any hidden infections (bacterial, viral, or both); address all hormonal imbalances; and tend to adrenal health.

I also want to say that stress and significant life events can serve as triggers for beginning to not feel well. Many friends of mine whom I have helped push to diagnosis say, "Ever since [my divorce, my surgery, my father's death, etc.], I haven't felt well."

Here is a list of the most common triggers related to the etiology of hypothyroid disease. Remember that autoimmune thyroid disease may have the same triggers, but the gut must be addressed and inflammation quelled in order to drive thyroid antibodies packing.

Mental/emotional/spiritual

- Caring for a chronically ill family member
- Divorce
- Death in the family
- Loss of a job
- Promotion that brings with it more responsibility
- Financial loss

Physical

- Autoimmune attack that targets the thyroid (Hashimoto's or Graves')
- Leaky gut
- Gluten allergy
- Whiplash or car accident
- Direct trauma to the thyroid, such as surgeries in the cervical area
- Radiation to the head and neck, especially in childhood

Chemical

- Low estrogen and testosterone at the time of menopause
- Low levels of selenium, zinc, and iodine
- Pollutants that interfere with thyroid hormone function, such as pesticides and PCBs

LEARN TO SPOT THE SIGNS

So something triggers thyroid failure, and that manifests itself in outward symptoms. Let's review those symptoms one more time. In the early stages of thyroid malfunction, you may experience:

- Weakness
- Fatigue
- Cold intolerance
- Joint and muscle pain

- Paleness
- Thin and brittle fingernails
- Depression
- Constipation

As months and years pass and you are not diagnosed or optimally treated, though, you may begin to experience:

- Slow speech
- Dry, flaky skin
- Thinning of your eyebrows
- Hoarseness
- Abnormal menstrual periods
- Puffy face, hands, and feet
- Thickening of your skin
- Decreased ability to taste and smell

It's important for you to learn these signs so you can help not only yourself but also others in your life who may be victims of thyroid malfunction and disease.

It is heartbreaking to watch a person's life be impacted by the negative effects of thyroid disease. This is particularly true for a young woman, as symptoms seem to rear their ugly head or become worse during puberty or after pregnancy. These symptoms are very distressing to a young woman because they affect everything about her endocrine system when she is just becoming aware of what her endocrine system is for.

She may notice that her friends can enjoy a very active life both socially and physically, often running or walking several miles per day and/or going to CrossFit, spin class, or just about anything their vibrant health and strong bodies care to do.

But to a young girl or woman who begins a decline due to hypothyroidism during the prepubescent years and beyond, life can be a series of letdowns. While her friends are running, all she may want to do is sleep during the day while suffering with insomnia as she lies awake at night. She may feel depressed and alone while her friends are grabbing all of what life has to offer.

Her weight begins to climb even though her dietary habits are not any different than those of her friends. She knows girls that can eat just about anything they want without gaining a single pound.

When her friends are active and enjoying life, she often finds herself battling a lingering cold, flu, throat infection, or virus. When she does push herself to "run with her friends," she finds that she pays a price: exhaustion from which she takes days to recover.

Her friends may complain of PMS, but she will have PMS symptoms that are off the charts. She may deal with heavy, irregular periods, anxiety, depression, and body aches that are very different from those suffered by her friends with healthy thyroid function.

She will often deal with polycystic ovary syndrome (PCOS), blood sugar–handling problems, or insulin resistance, otherwise known as metabolic syndrome. Her hair may thin as her friends are excited about going to the salon to experiment with the latest color, Brazilian blowouts, and keratin treatments. While her friends are thriving, she may begin sprouting dark hair in places that are typically male in pattern.

So her parents take her to the doctor. Where does she

begin with such a litany of life-disrupting and embarrassing complaints?

The family doctor will run the standard tests: CBC (complete blood chemistry), iron, TSH (thyroid-stimulating hormone), glucose, A1C (this measures your blood sugar control over the past two to three months), and metabolic profile. What will he be able to tell from these tests? When an underlying hypothyroid issue is involved, the total cholesterol will be higher than normal, with lipids (blood fats) as well as triglycerides often in a zone that is entirely too high, which can be a sign of blood sugar imbalance. In addition, her glucose reading may be high even though her diet is not sugar laden. An astute doctor may find the culprit early, thus sparing a young woman years of poor health and even poorer quality of life.

Her heart rate may be slow, her body temperature and blood pressure low, and her reflexes sluggish, but the doctor may not chalk it up to anything. "She's young, and that body temp, low blood pressure, fatigue, and weight gain can be resolved by getting up and out. She's a woman now and needs to learn how to deal with her hormones. It's a 'woman thing.' Nothing major is showing up, and I am sure that stress is a factor." Unless the TSH is high, underlying thyroid disease may never be found. This is especially true when the underlying thyroid issue is autoimmune, since tests for thyroid antibodies are not generally run by most physicians the first time out. This one omission cost me, my girls, and untold other women *years* of quality of life.

How many young women have heard this? I was one of the unlucky ones, and so were both of my girls. Since our diagnoses, I have helped almost four hundred women and their precious daughters get to their diagnoses sooner instead of spending decades with life-disrupting symptoms being chalked up to just "being a woman."

My life's mission is to help you recognize the signs early that point to the root of your distress—hypothyroidism or autoimmune thyroiditis, otherwise known as Hashimoto's disease. Stealthier than a stealth bomber, thyroid disease can decimate your health!

It's More Than Just Stress

What prompted me to seek out help? What were my signs?

At first I complained of being fatigued and my muscles feeling heavy. My hair was coarse, I gained weight, my skin was dry, and my anxiety became worse. I really enjoyed the times when I could just rest with a warm, comfy blanket and my woolly, soft socks. I also found myself becoming less motivated and starting to decline or make up excuses when friends asked me to an event. My father passed away rather suddenly at the time, and it affected me greatly. Everyone around me said it must be grief. My son also went away to college that year, and there were several serious family issues going on that were very upsetting. All of this, plus a writing career, made a diagnosis of stress easy.

Little did I know that I had been dealing with an autoimmune thyroid issue most of my life. My lifelong subnormal body temperature of 96.8 was a big clue, as were the frequent infections and the inability to handle stress without getting sick afterward. These issues should have tipped someone off that I had not only a thyroid issue but also exhausted adrenals. But again, you will rarely meet a conventional practitioner who makes the thyroid-adrenal connection.

The problem for my daughters and me was that it took years to find all of this out. We were given thyroid medication only and told to take vitamin D. We still felt awful. This was only peeling the top layer of this very big onion—only now I realized it was going to be up to me to peel the rest.

How to Get Your Diagnosis

If you are going to see your family practitioner, simply relay your list of symptoms to him or her. Ask for a thyroid panel to be done. I am sure your doctor will have no objection to this.

In addition, you need to ask your doctor to order a TPO (thyroid peroxidase antibody) test and a TgAb (thyroglobulin antibody) test to check for antibodies. If you have any antibodies, you have autoimmune thyroid disease. This is true even if your TSH is normal—I repeat, even if your TSH is normal!

I was undiagnosed for forty years because no one looked for antibodies. This one test can help save you from years of going from one specialist to another, trying to find the cause of your plethora of symptoms that seem to compound with each decade of life. Remember, most cases of hypothyroidism are autoimmune or Hashimoto's thyroiditis, and the treatment for autoimmune thyroid disease is not as straightforward as the treatment for hypothyroidism.

If you are found to have antibodies, you have to address the trigger that is causing your body to launch an attack upon your thyroid. Many studies show a strong link between wheat gluten and Hashimoto's.[2] When my daughters and I were tested for anti-gliadin antibodies, the results came back showing high antibodies to gluten. Gliadin is the portion of gluten that causes an immune reaction (antibodies) in certain individuals, such as those with celiac disease and Hashimoto's. This meant that the real underlying problem was our immune systems rather than only our thyroid glands.

If you have the thyroid blood test panel run, complete with TPO and TgAb, and your test shows that you do have antibodies, the next step is to do a stool test and/or serum (blood) test for gliadin antibodies, which are so common to Hashimoto's. If your results are positive, get the gluten and all grains out of your life. Autoimmunity begins in the gut. You can't get well with an inflamed gut. Gluten inflames not only the gut but also the skin, joints, brain, and respiratory tract. Once you find out that you have antibodies to gluten, you must avoid it for life. (I will address all these things in later chapters.)

To review, getting to your diagnosis means taking the following steps:

1. Make a list of your symptoms.
2. List any account of thyroid disease in your family history.
3. Have your physician do a "hands-on" examination of your neck. This is wise to do, but it does not always aid in finding small abnormalities. It is only a starting point.
4. Get a standard thyroid panel run, but make sure your doctor adds in TPO and TgAb.
5. If your TSH is high, get thyroid medication and support.
6. If your antibodies and TSH are high, eliminate gluten and take thyroid medication.
7. Find out if you have a gluten intolerance. You may order a test from EnteroLab (www.enterolab.com) that will inform you if you have a genetic predisposition for gluten

intolerance. They recommend avoiding gluten forever if your test comes back positive.

Concerning the blood work, here is a more detailed breakdown of the panels and tests you want your doctor to run:

- TSH: This is considered the most sensitive measure of thyroid status and used as a benchmark for the management of hypothyroidism and thyroid cancer care. Now researchers are suggesting that additional markers must be more closely evaluated in the ongoing management of thyroid disease.[3]
- Free T4: Measures thyroid hormone available to enter cells.
- T3: Measures total T3 (another thyroid hormone).
- Free T3: Measures "unbound" T3.
- Reverse T3 (RT3): Measures reverse T3, an inactive product of T4 that increases during illness and stress. What happens if you make too much RT3? It will become an issue. It binds to the T3 receptor sites, which blocks the beneficial effects of T3, and the result is that you remain functionally hypothyroid and have many of the lingering symptoms even if your labs look normal.

  Many people who have to constantly adjust their thyroid hormone medication have T3 thyroid hormone resistance. Typically a patient with thyroid hormone resistance will begin on one dose and have to continually increase the dosage because they feel good for a few weeks and then their symptoms return. This continual need for dose increase is a sure sign of thyroid resistance syndrome. It usually is resolved with T3-only therapy at least until RT3 levels remain in the acceptable range.

- Thyroglobulin (TG): Measures thyroglobulin, a unique protein from thyroid cells, a marker for Hashimoto's thyroiditis and important in thyroid cancer care and management.
- TPO antibody: Measures autoimmunity in thyroid disease such as Hashimoto's disease and Graves' disease.
- Thyroglobulin antibody (TgAb): Measures autoimmunity to thyroglobulin for Hashimoto's disease and is a thyroid cancer marker for follow-up care.
- Thyroid-stimulating immunoglobulin (TSI): Measures autoimmune antibody to TSH receptor for Graves' disease.
- Ultrasound: I highly recommend a baseline ultrasound of your thyroid gland. This is especially true if you have been found to have TPO and/or TgAb in your blood. This means that you do, in fact, have an autoimmune thyroid disease and that there is an inflammatory attack by your own body causing damage to your thyroid gland. Often you will have nodules from the inflammation.

> I like to use the comparison of an oyster. Do you know how pearls are formed? A tiny bit of sand gets inside the oyster, and in time the irritation, or inflammation, from that tiny bit of sand causes a pearl to form. Apply this to your thyroid—inflammation causes a nodule to form within the thyroid. Nodules do form in hypothyroidism without autoimmune involvement.
>
> I recommend that you keep a folder of your thyroid ultrasound reports. I used these reports to monitor my nodule's growth and characteristic changes after my Hashimoto's diagnosis.

If you are a thyroid patient, you should be aware that it is very common to have vitamin and mineral deficiencies. It is imperative to keep track of your B_{12}, vitamin D, iron and/or ferritin levels. A deficit in any one of these can affect the way your body utilizes thyroid hormone. I recommend that you ask to have these levels tested each time you visit your doctor, as it is crucial for ideal management of your condition. Since adrenal issues can adversely affect the way your body coverts T4 to T3, I also suggest having your a.m. and p.m. cortisol levels tested. And since all of our hormones work together in symphony, you should also have your sex hormone levels checked routinely. Sex hormone abnormalities often pop up when thyroid hormone function is low.

Here is your guide to the important tests that will help you and your health-care provider manage your thyroid health:[4]

- Comprehensive metabolic profile (CMP): This test will measure your glucose levels, electrolyte and fluid balance, kidney function, and liver function. This is important for assessing your general chemical balance and metabolism.
- Complete blood count (CBC): A common test that will assess the type and number of cells in your blood, especially red blood cells, white blood cells, and platelets. It may help to diagnose conditions such as anemia and infection that are found often in autoimmune thyroid issues as well as many other disorders.
- Vitamin D_3 (25-hydroxyvitamin D): Crucial to a properly functioning immune system, vitamin D is especially important for thyroid patients because autoimmune thyroid disease is the most common cause of an under- or overactive thyroid. Research shows that patients deficient in vitamin D are more likely to have elevated thyroid antibody tests and are prone to autoimmunity in general. Optimal levels should be between 50 and 80 ng/mL.[5]
- Vitamin B_{12}: You should be aware that there is an association between autoimmune thyroid disease and B_{12} deficiency, and up to 40 percent of hypothyroid patients are deficient. Many symptoms of vitamin B_{12} deficiency can overlap with thyroid disease, which can make it difficult to distinguish the symptoms. Normal B_{12} values are typically 200–900 pg/mL, but new evidence suggests that optimal

levels should be near the top of the range, or over 600 pg/mL.[6]

- Iron (percentage of saturation, TIBC, and serum iron): Iron is vital in thyroid hormone synthesis. It is important to note that autoimmune thyroid patients have a high incidence of iron deficiency. That is why I recommend that women who are anemic have their thyroid checked as soon as possible. Many people with anemia that has been hard to manage have thyroid issues that have yet to be unmasked. Total iron-binding capacity (TIBC) measures the amount of protein available to transport iron. Normal ranges are 240–450 mcg/dL. Iron saturation measures the saturation of the proteins that transport iron. Normal ranges are between 20 and 50 percent. Serum iron measures the iron level in your blood. Normal levels range from 60 to 170 mcg/dL.[7]
- Ferritin: Having your ferritin levels checked is very important, as it is the major iron storage protein of the body. If you have unexplained fatigue and your ferritin levels are below 50 micrograms per milliliter, you should be considered for iron supplementation. Ferritin levels for women should be closer to 70–90, while levels for men should be near 100–110.[8]
- Cortisol: This is a big one! It is now becoming more well known (especially among functional medicine physicians) that adrenal dysfunction often accompanies thyroid issues. The thyroid

and the adrenal glands work together; when one of them is underperforming, it is certain that the other will be running on a deficit. When cortisol levels are not optimal, thyroid hormone cannot be utilized properly and vice versa. Many doctors do not factor this in, and it can cause years of unsatisfactory care. Ask for the twenty-four-hour saliva cortisol/DHEA test to evaluate adrenal function. It is an excellent test for detecting low cortisol levels, and it gives a more complete picture than a single cortisol blood test.

- Sex hormone panel: As I mentioned earlier, hormones are interrelated and act in symphony. If one hormone level is not optimal, this affects other hormone levels. Many functional medicine practitioners prefer saliva testing, but blood tests are also common. You should know that untreated thyroid disease can often lead to "hormonal hades," causing excess testosterone, low testosterone, low progesterone/estrogen dominance, and symptoms or conditions such as polycystic ovary syndrome, low libido, infertility, endometriosis, and more.

THIS IS A LONG PATH

When you have an invisible disease such as Hashimoto's, you might look OK on the outside and your appearance might look put together. People may not really grasp that it's an "inside job" that

- levels you with depression while it amps you with anxiety;

- slows you to a halt;
- fogs your brain;
- disrupts your speech and cohesive thoughts;
- leaves you unable to function enough to put a menu plan together
  or take a trip to the grocery store
  or clean up the house
  or drive on the freeway
  or handle bright lights, loud noise, fast movements, or certain foods
  All because you feel as though you were hit by a truck.

Chances are you will encounter all of this and more if you aren't educated on these manifestations of thyroid disease and how to take care of yourself. But you are now wiser than many of the physicians you will seek out for treatment. Because of this you will get to a diagnosis sooner and also have a better chance at receiving the proper treatment.

Now let's turn to the more specific ways thyroid disease can wreak havoc on our lives. To be forewarned is to be forearmed!

It has been widely reported in the media that Elizabeth Taylor suffered from more than seventy illnesses and serious injuries. She was born with scoliosis, which may be associated with thyroid conditions.[9] Throughout her life she experienced hospitalizations and surgeries that included an appendectomy, tracheotomy, crushed spinal discs, skin cancer, and various other issues. In addition to having both hips replaced, she also had a brain tumor removed, suffered from congestive heart failure, struggled with weight issues, and had constant pain from her back injuries. This led to abuse of prescription painkillers and alcohol, and by her own admission, claims to have nearly died on four different occasions.[10]

Keep in mind that other heart problems and diseases can contribute to heart failure, such as congenital heart disease, heart attack, heart valve disease, arrhythmias, emphysema, severe anemia, and thyroid problems.[11]

Notice the long list of severely stressful and painful events in Liz Taylor's life. I am sure her adrenal glands were weakened. Notice the infections, both bacterial and viral. Notice the mention of *seventy* illnesses.

Also note that this article talks about congestive heart failure as the cause of Elizabeth Taylor's death. As I will prove in a later chapter, hypothyroidism can be the root cause of congestive heart failure, and it can progress until it is the "last stop" on the bus ride of life.

Let's take a look at Elizabeth Taylor's long and painful struggle with health issues and emotional turmoil before that fateful last diagnosis. Consider this: there is a direct correlation between congestive heart failure and thyroid disease.[12] That is tragic, and in my opinion it strengthens my point that we must PUSH.

In Elizabeth's era few physicians knew the far-reaching effects of undiagnosed and undertreated thyroid disease. In addition, Elizabeth experienced painful injuries, many surgeries, and much heartbreak in her life that surely taxed her adrenal glands to the point of sheer exhaustion. As a matter of fact, she did suffer from bouts of exhaustion and actually collapsed from stress in 1953.[13]

After reading many biographies of Elizabeth Taylor, I personally believe that her constitution was weakened from an early age. In her later years she was quoted as saying, "I enter hospitals as often as others enter taxi cabs."[14]

Her many rounds of antibiotics affected her gut's terrain, causing her to have leaky gut and, no doubt, autoimmune issues, judging by the list of symptoms. You can see that she had most of the hypothyroid symptoms and conditions that are mentioned in this book. Remember that hypothyroidism can contribute greatly to the development of high cholesterol and atherosclerosis, which can lead to congestive heart failure.

Could an underlying thyroid issue have caused her to suffer so many infections and so much angst? Could her alcohol and painkiller addictions have been caused by her inability to cope with her physical and emotional pain—pain that is so common, by the way, with adrenal exhaustion? Could her marriages have failed due to her inability to recover emotionally from her husband Mike Todd's tragic death? Note that because of an illness, she was unable to join him on the fateful day when he died in a plane crash.

This constellation of illnesses and stress reactions all point to hypothyroidism and low adrenal function earlier rather than later in life. Could Elizabeth Taylor have been spared much agony by having the right thyroid tests run? Take a look at this time line of her life as reported online:[15]

1944 Suffered a concussion and back injuries while filming *National Velvet*

1951 Divorced Nicky Hilton Jr.

1953 Collapsed because of stress and back problems; had to have surgery to remove flint from her eye; gave birth to a son by cesarean

1955 Got influenza, had to have blood transfusions; suffered from sciatica; hospitalized for pinched nerve and flu; gave birth to her second son by cesarean

1956 Endured a five-hour spinal operation to repair crushed disks

1957 When her daughter was born prematurely, had birth complications; had a tubal ligation to prevent further pregnancies; also had an appendectomy; divorced Michael Wilding (they had gotten married in 1952)

1958 Husband Mike Todd died in a plane crash—she would have been on the plane had she not been at home ill (they had married in 1957)

1959 Had double pneumonia and tonsillitis

1960 Fell on a patch of ice and broke her leg; had to have oral surgery for gum abscess; while filming *Cleopatra*, contracted a viral illness

1961 Developed viral pneumonia and a lung infection, which necessitated a tracheotomy; was given an hour to live after a lung collapsed; developed a leg infection caused by intravenous feeding; had plastic surgery to remove the tracheotomy scar

1962 After resuming the filming of *Cleopatra*, got food poisoning—rumored to be a suicide attempt/overdose after a fight with Richard Burton

1963 Had surgery on her leg and knee

1964 Divorced Eddie Fisher (they had gotten married in 1959); suffered back and arm injuries from being mobbed by fans

1966 Broke a toe while making *The Taming of the Shrew*

1969 Had a hysterectomy; that same year was in traction with more back issues

1971 Had a cyst below her right eye removed

1973 Had surgery to remove an ovarian cyst; was quarantined with measles in Italy

1974 Divorced Richard Burton (they had been married since 1964)

1975 Contracted amoebic dysentery

1976 Fell from a horse, aggravating her existing back problems; divorced Burton again (they had remarried in 1975)

1977 Hospitalized for back problems; broke finger in a sledding accident

1978 At a dinner event, choked on a chicken bone and was rushed to the hospital; had surgery to remove metal dust from right eye; also broke wrist, twisted ankle tripping over a carpet, and was hospitalized for pneumonia

1979 Had oral surgery; fell and broke a rib

1980 Hospitalized for infected sinuses

1981 Had severe cases of laryngitis and bronchitis; was rushed to the hospital after a heart attack scare; broke arm while skiing

1982 Sent to the hospital for a respiratory infection; divorced John Warner (they had married in 1976)

1983 Injured a leg and her neck in car crash; was hospitalized after eating a spoiled taco; got bronchitis and laryngitis again

1984 Went to the Betty Ford Center for addictions to painkillers and alcohol

1985 Was injured while filming *North and South* and had to be hospitalized; was stricken with food poisoning

1986 Twisted her neck and had to wear a surgical collar; was hospitalized for complications from a root canal

1987 Damaged her knee after falling on the Swiss ski slopes

1988 Was hospitalized for back pain

1989 Again was hospitalized for back pain; returned to Betty Ford

1990 Contracted viral pneumonia, bacterial pneumonia, and a yeast infection in her mouth, and had to have a lung biopsy

1996 Divorced Larry Fortensky (they had married in 1991)

1997 Had brain surgery to remove a benign mass from the lining of her frontal lobe

1998 Fell on her sixty-sixth birthday and had to be hospitalized for bruises and hip and back injuries

1999 Broke a bone in her back in a fall

2000 Contracted pneumonia; it is discovered that she had an enlarged heart—a sign of thyroid disease[16]

2009 Had heart surgery

2011 Died of congestive heart failure

With increased awareness about thyroid disease among Hollywood's elite, more and more stories about their experiences and struggles with this energy-zapping condition have come to light. Some of the most popular celebrities of our time have experienced thyroid cancer and have taken up the cause of increasing thyroid disease awareness.

Gena Lee Nolin, *Baywatch* star, experienced fatigue, weight gain, and other issues in each of her pregnancies and was told that she simply had a case of postpartum depression. In 2008 she discovered that she had Hashimoto's disease and hypothyroidism.[17]

Actress and thyroid cancer survivor Sofia Vergara successfully battled thyroid cancer in 2002. She told *Parade* magazine, "I've been through it all, so I don't take life's little dramas too seriously. I say, don't sweat the small stuff, because there's bigger stuff that can really make you sweat."[18]

Actress Catherine Bell (*JAG*, *Army Wives*, *The Good Witch*) is yet another thyroid cancer survivor.[19]

Kim Cattrall, best known for her role in *Sex in the City*, deals with Hashimoto's disease.[20] Cattrall is over fifty and at the age when women most commonly develop thyroid conditions.

Tipper Gore, wife of former vice president Al Gore, had a benign thyroid tumor that required her to have half of her thyroid removed in 1999.[21]

Multi-Grammy-winner Linda Ronstadt is yet another

celebrity that has reportedly struggled with hypothyroidism for many years.[22]

What rock star Rod Stewart thought to be a benign vocal nodule was later revealed to be cancer, a slow-growing papillary thyroid carcinoma. In May 2001 he had surgery at Cedars-Sinai Medical Center in Los Angeles to have his thyroid gland removed, and he feared that he would lose his singing voice. Thankfully he regained his voice, made a full recovery, and is now committed to raising awareness about the disease.[23]

Chapter 4

THYROID CANCER

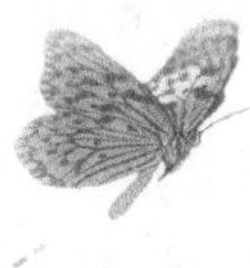

AFTER MY DAUGHTERS and I were diagnosed with Hashimoto's thyroiditis, we were given thyroid pills and sent on our way. "Not so fast," I argued. Having done my research on autoimmune disease, I knew that it always involved inflammation. I also knew that inflammation sets the stage for all kinds of degenerative diseases, including cancer.

I demanded an ultrasound but was told, "Oh, they won't find anything—just a ragged thyroid from the autoimmune attack—so it isn't worth the trouble." I accepted that answer for five years as I became sicker and my daughters suffered with symptoms that made their young lives miserable.

One day I'd had enough pushback from the "top docs" in Arizona. Two of these physicians had written best-selling books on thyroid disease. I trusted them. After spending five years and most of my savings, I found a new doctor, who was actually an older doctor close to retirement. I thought he would help, as he was as close to the "good old family doctor" as I could find.

He was a breath of fresh air. He listened to me and said, "Of course, I think an ultrasound is a very wise thing to do." And with that order in my hand, I was scanned.

The results? A nodule. It was solitary, with characteristics that made it suspicious—it had microcalcifications. Not a good characteristic to have in a nodule. But it was only 4 mm in size, so they said I was OK and told me to watch it.

I was so involved with my daughters' declining health that much time passed. We all continued to get worse, and it was compounded by the death of my mother, the move far away from my hometown, and the breakup of my thirty-four-year marriage.

As my youngest daughter continued to get worse, I got worse too, and was paralyzed by the trauma of it all. My adrenal glands were completely worn out, and I couldn't push anymore. I was in trouble.

By the grace of God I got my wits and my determination back and took my youngest daughter to the same family doctor who had agreed to have me scanned. He took one look at her neck after we went over the long list of symptoms and said, "Mama, I see that her neck is not symmetrical. Let's get her scanned."

The next day she was scanned, and the following day the phone rang—the doctor said, "Mama, we've got a problem. Your girl has thyroid cancer, and it's all over her thyroid."

I asked what to do next.

He said, "You're smart. Do your homework, and find a good surgeon. Get a biopsy, and get that thyroid out."

I was dumbfounded. How could this be happening? Was this a bad dream? "Do my homework"? Wasn't that why I took her to a doctor?

Know Your Nodules

Let's begin by looking at what a thyroid nodule really is. It is a growth or mass in the thyroid gland that is not the same as healthy thyroid tissue. The doctor often detects a nodule when she feels it during a physical exam. Even if the doctor cannot detect a nodule, one may still exist, as some can only be found by ultrasound or CAT scan.

Most thyroid nodules are not cancerous. In fact, only about 5 to 10 percent are malignant.[1] The majority of nodules that are not malignant could be best described as cysts, which are filled with fluid. In a person with an overactive thyroid gland, this condition can promote a benign tumor, and these tumors rarely become cancerous. If a suspicious nodule is found during the examination, the doctor will try to determine whether it lends itself to malignancy by using standard procedures that include blood tests, ultrasound imaging, or a fine-needle aspiration (FNA) biopsy. Keep in mind that most doctors do not like to biopsy nodules that are smaller than one centimeter, preferring to watch them for growth or suspicious changes by periodic ultrasound. I feel it is important to tell you here that my papillary thyroid cancer was found in a solitary nodule that was only seven millimeters in diameter. The only clue that showed the radiologist that it was malignant was the presence of microcalcifications within the nodule.

My and my youngest daughter's nodules were small but worrisome, so I sought out a radiologist to perform an ultrasound biopsy.

During the biopsy my neck was tilted way back, and the radiologist used a tiny needle, smaller than the needle normally used for drawing blood, to numb the skin over the nodule with lidocaine. Once I was numb, he put the needle into my nodule several times to extract a little tissue fluid with some thyroid cells into the barrel of the needle. The experience was not pleasant, but it was not too uncomfortable either. The cell samples were put onto a glass slide and sent to the pathology department.

In my case two different radiologists reviewed my

ultrasound results for five years. One of them said my nodule was suspicious due to characteristics that matched those commonly found in papillary thyroid cancer. He reassured me that it was a very small nodule, though, and that since papillary thyroid cancer is slow growing, it warranted watching only; its four-millimeter size created no sense of urgency. In the five years of observation it grew from four millimeters to seven millimeters. I knew it was time to push my doctor hard even though it was still small. What I have learned since then is that there are microcancers smaller than one centimeter that can go undetected, as was true in my case. These cancers can be aggressive even though they are small.

The Path Through Pathology

When a biopsy is performed and the results are in, the pathologist may report finding nothing but blood on the slide. Ten to fifteen percent of FNA biopsies result in what is referred to as an *inadequate specimen*,[2] but just because nothing was found doesn't mean there is nothing to find. The test should be repeated until a sample can be evaluated and it can be determined whether the nodule is benign or malignant. Even if the biopsy finds that the nodule appears to be noncancerous, in a very small percentage of cases it can still become cancerous. This is referred to as a false-negative biopsy. For this reason patients who undergo biopsies of this nature need to be reexamined, which may include an FNA biopsy, every six to twelve months.[3]

The thyroid ultrasound test is an important diagnostic tool that is also periodically done in both the discovery and management of thyroid nodules. If the ultrasound finds that the nodule is growing or that new nodules are present, a repeat biopsy should be ordered. This should also be the approach if abnormal lymph nodes are found or begin to grow. If the nodule doesn't change over time, it should be watched, but another biopsy isn't needed until something suspicious necessitates it.

The pathologist becomes a very valuable partner in the whole discovery process. In his lab he can see if there are changes in cells that, while they might not indicate cancer, may be suspect and are not normal in benign nodules. This is a marker called *atypia of undetermined significance* or *follicular lesion of undetermined significance*. It doesn't necessarily conclude anything, but the observation is enough to recommend that the biopsy be repeated.

Just as there is a result called a false-negative, there can also be a false-positive result, when a pathologist reports that the biopsy is suspicious for cancer when it is actually benign. This occurs in a small percentage of cases. Typically, when a false-positive occurs, surgery is performed to allow greater examination of the tissue to know for sure and to treat the cancerous thyroid, if that turns out to be the case.

In some cases a nodule is determined to be a tumor but the pathologist can't determine if it is benign or cancerous. Although only 20 to 30 percent of these tumors are indeed cancerous, the safest approach is to remove the thyroid gland.

Why Do Nodules Develop?

There are five main precipitators that cause thyroid nodules.

1. Iodine deficiency

A lack of iodine in your diet can cause your thyroid gland to develop thyroid nodules. This is very uncommon in the United States, as iodine is routinely added to table salt and other foods. But you should know that without adequate iodine intake, your thyroid gland can progressively enlarge and develop a goiter in an attempt to keep up with the demand for thyroid hormone production. It is also important for you to know that nodules can develop within a goiter. A person who develops a large goiter may experience symptoms of choking, especially when lying down, and have difficulty swallowing and breathing. This is more common in third world countries, however, where there is a greater chance of low iodine intake.

2. Overgrowth of thyroid tissue

Sometimes normal thyroid tissue overgrows for reasons that are not clearly understood. This overgrowth of thyroid tissue is referred to as a thyroid adenoma. The good news here is that thyroid adenomas are benign, or noncancerous. A thyroid adenoma may, however, become a problem simply because of its size. It can also become a problem if it produces thyroid hormones on its own. This overproduction of thyroid hormones directly contributes to hyperthyroidism.

3. Thyroid cyst

Thyroid nodules can also be caused by fluid-filled cavities called cysts. Cysts most commonly result from degenerating thyroid adenomas. Occasionally the fluid in thyroid cysts is mixed with solid components, and while these cysts are usually benign, the solid components can be malignant. This was true in my youngest daughter's case. This is why you *must* be vigilant to be aware of changes in any nodule, whether it be an adenoma, a cyst, or an enlarged thyroid gland.

4. Chronic inflammation

My daughters and I lived with this condition for decades without diagnosis. Chronic lymphocytic thyroiditis, otherwise known as Hashimoto's disease, causes chronic inflammation of the thyroid and is another cause of nodules. It can also cause thyroid inflammation that causes nodules to grow over time. Hashimoto's is an autoimmune disease that results in the slow destruction of your thyroid gland. It is often marked with periods of reduced thyroid gland activity (hypothyroidism) and periods of increased thyroid activity (hyperthyroidism) until the gland is rendered completely unable to produce enough thyroid hormone for optimal health.

5. Cancer

A nodule can indeed be thyroid cancer. It is generally believed that the chances of a nodule being malignant are small. My daughter and I were reassured many times after our ultrasounds and biopsies that we were just fine! We were told that people just don't get cancer in a nodule if they have Hashimoto's disease. They were wrong!

Here are the risk factors commonly associated with the development of thyroid cancer:

- Family history of thyroid or other endocrine cancers
- Age—older than thirty and younger than sixty are at greater risk
- Gender—men have a higher risk
- History of radiation exposure, especially in childhood, particularly to the head and neck

My daughter and I did not have the risk factors, so there was no sense of alarm—until the last biopsy, which indeed revealed papillary cancer!

PUSH! Make sure you do your homework; fire your doctor, hire a new one—do whatever it takes to make sure your thyroid is not harboring a cancerous nodule.

Remember these key points about thyroid nodules:

- They are lumps that develop in a gland that is often otherwise healthy.
- Nodules frequently grow in the edges of the thyroid.
- Depending on their location, they can feel like a lump in the throat, or they can appear as a lump in the neck.
- Some thyroid nodules are cysts filled with fluid.
- One in twelve young women develops a thyroid nodule.
- One in forty young men has a thyroid nodule.
- Fifty percent of all people aged fifty will have a thyroid nodule.
- Sixty percent of all people aged sixty will have a thyroid nodule.
- Seventy percent of all people aged seventy will have a thyroid nodule.
- Ninety-five percent of all thyroid nodules are benign.

Given these statistics and knowing what I know now due to actually having experienced thyroid cancer, I feel it is wise to have your thyroid checked by ultrasound at least once at the beginning of each decade of life starting at puberty. If a nodule is found, you should have it monitored and/or biopsied as long or as many times as it takes to get a definitive diagnosis. I kept my scans in a folder and noted the growth, albeit small, over the course of several years. I noted the changes and pushed from ultrasound to biopsy to surgery to recovery. You must be proactive.

Four Types of Thyroid Cancer

While it is common to have a thyroid nodule and to have some disease issues that cause varying levels of malfunction of the gland, these conditions seldom manifest as thyroid cancer. For unknown reasons the occurrence of thyroid cancer is on the rise. This could be in part to more routine screenings of thyroid glands than ever before or it may have an environmental causation. The treatments for thyroid cancer are usually effective, especially when the cancer is found early. Thyroid cancer has a variety of forms, and some are more dangerous than others. But the most common are fortunately the most treatable. Once thyroid cancer has been discovered and effectively treated, however, caution is still required, because it is known to reoccur, often many years after the treatment.

What causes thyroid cancer?

There is no direct known cause for thyroid cancer; however, there are markers that seem to point to a higher incidence of the disease. DNA seems to play a role, so family history and certain events that can affect the DNA seem to be a link. Some scientists believe that radiation can play a role in causing the disease. There is also suspicion that childhood radiation treatment of the head, neck, and chest may have had a role. It is advisable to reduce your exposure to radiation and excessive X-rays, if possible. The occasional dental X-ray does not seem to be harmful, but people in high-risk groups may want to ask their dentists for a special collar that shields the thyroid from exposure. If you have had thyroid cancer, you should insist on it, as I always do.

It is important to be familiar with the symptoms of thyroid cancer. These symptoms may or may not occur together, and some people do not have any symptoms at all.

- The feeling of a lump or swelling in the neck
- A consistent pain in the front of the neck, which may include the ears
- Difficulty swallowing
- Restricted breathing, or wheezing
- A hoarse voice
- A frequent cough not related to a cold

Thyroid cancer is most commonly found by a doctor finding a lump or nodule in the neck during a routine examination. Any lump or nodule found is cause to look further and determine its nature. If there is any question, a biopsy should be performed to check for cancer cells. Once cancer is determined by the pathologist, he or she will identify which of the four types of thyroid cancer it is.

1. Papillary thyroid cancer

My daughter and I shared this diagnosis. This is the most common type of thyroid cancer and makes up 70 to 80 percent of all thyroid cancers. Papillary thyroid cancer is commonly diagnosed between the ages of thirty and fifty. Women are affected three times more often than men. This cancer usually is not aggressive, but it may spread, although usually not beyond the neck. Papillary tumor development is believed to be connected to radiation exposure, especially radiation treatments for adenoid problems or acne in childhood.[4]

2. Follicular thyroid cancer

Follicular cancer is often diagnosed between the ages of forty and sixty and makes up about 10 to 15 percent of all thyroid cancers. Again, women are affected three times more often than men. Unlike papillary thyroid cancer, follicular thyroid cancer cells may invade blood vessels and travel to other body parts such as bone or lung tissues. In addition, this cancer can be more aggressive in older patients.[5]

3. Medullary thyroid cancer

Medullary thyroid cancer is more likely to run in families and is associated with other endocrine disorders. It makes up about 5 to 10 percent of all thyroid cancers. It develops in the cells that produce calcitonin, which regulates calcium and promotes bone growth. An elevated calcitonin level can often be a cancer indicator. This type of thyroid cancer is often diagnosed between the ages of forty and fifty, and unlike papillary and follicular thyroid cancers, men and women are equally affected. The forms of medullary thyroid cancer include sporadic, which simply means not inherited; multiple endocrine neoplasia (MEN) types 1 and 2, which are genetic syndromes involving other parts of the endocrine system; and familial, meaning genetic but not linked to other MEN-related endocrine tumors.[6]

4. Anaplastic thyroid cancer—the least common thyroid cancer

Anaplastic thyroid cancer is very rare, affecting fewer than 5 percent of thyroid cancer patients. It requires aggressive treatment and is the most deadly of all thyroid cancers. Sadly many people who are diagnosed with anaplastic thyroid cancer do not live one year from the day they are diagnosed. It usually occurs in patients older than sixty-five, and women are affected more often than men. Unfortunately it is aggressive and invasive, and therefore it is the least responsive to treatment.[7]

Anaplastic thyroid cancer is usually treated with surgery if at all possible, and then with radioactive iodine (RAI). Radioactive iodine therapy is used to destroy remaining thyroid cells and thyroid cancer cells that remain after the thyroid gland has been removed. Radioactive iodine is usually given as a liquid or capsule that is swallowed. Unfortunately only a small number of anaplastic cancer patients are even candidates for surgical intervention in the hopes of catching it early enough to cure it. Usually doctors resort to more aggressive therapy such as external beam radiation or chemotherapy in an effort to save the life of the patient. But all too often the patient has experienced significant invasion to vital neck, lung, and bone structures, making the cancer inoperable even at the time of initial diagnosis.

Four Stages of Papillary Thyroid Cancer

If you have been diagnosed with the most common thyroid cancer, papillary thyroid cancer, the good news is that it rarely needs chemo or radiation therapy. The treatment you are assigned will depend on your age and the stage of your disease.

> **Stage 1.** In patients younger than forty-five, stage 1 means papillary thyroid cancer of any size is found in the thyroid gland but also may be present in nearby lymph nodes and/or tissue in the neck. At stage 1 the cancer has

not spread to distant sites. In patients forty-five years of age and older, stage 1 papillary cancer is usually located only in the thyroid gland, not in nearby neck tissue or lymph nodes, and is less than three-quarters of an inch. It has not spread to distant sites. This was my case; I was stage 1.

Stage 2. For a patient under the age of forty-five, stage 2 cancer has spread beyond the thyroid and neck area and can be metastasizing elsewhere. In patients forty-five or older, the cancer is in the thyroid only and has not spread to nearby neck tissue, lymph nodes, or other sites. At this stage it is one to one and a half inches in size.

Stage 3. In patients forty-five years of age and older, stage 3 papillary thyroid cancer means that either a cancerous tumor of any size has spread to nearby lymph nodes but not to other sites, or a tumor larger than four centimeters has only minimally spread to neck tissue and not to other sites. This is more rare in people under forty-five; however, my daughter had stage 3 papillary cancer at age twenty-six, with a BRAF gene mutation that made her case not typical and more aggressive.

Stage 4. Also rare in people under forty-five, stage 4 means that the cancer has extensively affected the neck tissue, including large blood vessels, or it has spread to other parts of the body, such as the lungs or bones.

> It is important for you to remember that these are general staging guidelines and each individual it just that: individual! No two cases are alike!

In my daughter's case, since she was diagnosed with stage 3 papillary thyroid cancer, RAI treatment was ordered to ablate (destroy) any thyroid cancer cells and tissue the surgeon left behind after removing her thyroid gland. In my case, my cancer was stage 1 and confined to the thyroid with no lymph node involvement, so I did not have to undergo RAI treatment after my thyroid removal surgery.

I feel it is very important here to remind you that it was the autoimmune disease Hashimoto's thyroiditis—not the thyroid cancer—that made both of us feel very ill for many years. We did not have any symptoms that would make us think our thyroid glands harbored cancer. That is why it is so important to have tests done that will help ensure your thyroid is clear and free of cancer.

Finding out my daughter had thyroid cancer was a shock. It was a bigger shock finding out she had thyroid cancer because we were told that people with Hashimoto's autoimmune thyroid disease never have nodules that become malignant. That inaccurate statement could have cost my daughter her life!

If you feel uncomfortable with the information your health-care provider has given you, remember to PUSH—Push Until Something Happens. You will have to be more educated than your doctor about thyroid disease. It can mean the difference between just surviving and thriving.

Chapter 5

THE THYROID AND ADRENALS

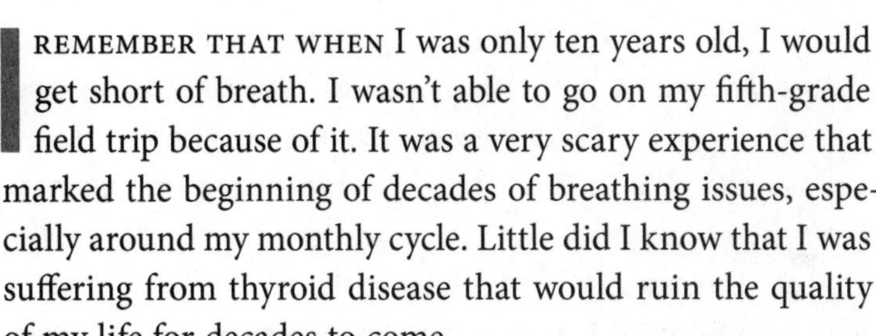

I REMEMBER THAT WHEN I was only ten years old, I would get short of breath. I wasn't able to go on my fifth-grade field trip because of it. It was a very scary experience that marked the beginning of decades of breathing issues, especially around my monthly cycle. Little did I know that I was suffering from thyroid disease that would ruin the quality of my life for decades to come.

In my forties, when I wrote books on natural healing, I found that taking the amino acid GABA helped to quell my shortness-of-breath issues that had escalated into full-blown panic attacks. When you can't breathe, you panic! While it gave me relief, it didn't address the underlying autoimmune thyroid condition that would not be diagnosed until years later. I flew across the country doing television shows and radio interviews and lectured at women's conferences, all while feeling as if I was losing ground with my own health. It was a devastating feeling to know that while I was helping others, I was declining.

The panic attacks became more intense after I moved to Arizona. Was it a coincidence? Or was my body running out of "life force"? I had always been a go-getter, a passionate woman, motivated to help heal the world, with energy to burn night and day. But now the anxiety and panic coupled with the yet-to-be-diagnosed Hashimoto's thyroiditis and major life changes had me on the sidelines of life.

I prayed for God to get me off the bench—but He had other plans.

THE ADRENAL STRIKE

What is important for you to remember, and as I have mentioned previously, your adrenal glands, your thyroid gland, and your gut's integrity are all interconnected. Your adrenal glands are part of your sympathetic nervous system. They secrete hormones such as epinephrine, norepinephrine, and cortisol—and believe me, these hormones are important to your well-being! They regulate your response to stress as well as your ability to even handle stress!

The million dollar question is whether an underperforming thyroid gland affects the adrenals, or if the adrenals are so taxed that they affect the thyroid gland. What we know for sure is that stress has a huge impact on your adrenal glands, and this in turn has a huge impact on the health of your thyroid. The big issue here is that stress creates a negative impact on your adrenal glands more than any other glands. And your adrenal gland response has a significant impact on your current and future state of health.

But stress alone does not tax your adrenal function. Many factors, such as blood sugar, leaky gut, food sensitivities (such as gluten sensitivity), food allergies, toxins, infections, inflammation, and autoimmune attacks (as with Hashimoto's thyroiditis, or any other autoimmune disease, for that matter), can cause your adrenal glands to release more stress hormones. This is why a holistic, proactive approach to your healing is so necessary. You simply cannot focus on one cause of adrenal stress without looking at the others.

The symptoms of adrenal stress are very similar to thyroid symptoms: fatigue, headaches, insomnia, mood swings, sugar and caffeine cravings, irritability, electrolyte imbalance, and dizziness. You'll find yourself struggling with how you react to stress or trauma, as well as dealing with changes in your body temperature, digestion, immune system, mood, libido, and energy levels. Why? Because adrenal stress can weaken your immunity, cause hormone imbalance, and disrupt the interaction between your adrenals and your other glands.

Adrenal stress also triggers your fight-or-flight response. Common activities such as standing in line at the grocery store, getting the kids ready for school in the morning, or even being asked to meet a friend for lunch might escalate quickly to high-alert status and trigger an anxiety attack. I experienced this for many years while not knowing my thyroid had exhausted my poor adrenals and my adrenals were functioning so poorly that autoimmunity set in on my dear thyroid gland.

Why does this happen? Because stress creates stress. That answer sounds simple, but it is complex. You experience external stress, and that triggers an internal stress response from your adrenals, and that stress response sends your sympathetic nervous system into attack mode. This chain reaction of stress in your body is the perfect storm that sets the stage for panic attacks. To put it another way, the more stress you experience, the less your adrenals can handle it, and the further you ride a downward spiral that can leave you unable to handle daily life.

In other words, adrenal stress and its resultant fatigue leave you situationally challenged. Brain fog, cloudy headedness, fatigue, sleep disruption, low blood pressure, lowered immune function, widespread inflammation, and low thyroid are all signs that point to low cortisol and underfunctioning, stressed adrenal glands.

How It Works

It is vitally important for you to know that low adrenal function can cause your thyroid issue to be much more intense than it would be otherwise. That is why some people with thyroid disease and adequate adrenal function simply take thyroid replacement hormone and do quite well, while others with underlying adrenal issues struggle for years wondering why their friends are doing well on thyroid hormone medication while they never seem to "turn a corner." Known as your life-saving organs that sit atop your kidneys, the adrenals, when working at full speed, help to make life a wonderful experience. They secrete many of your most important hormones, including pregnenolone, adrenaline, estrogen, progesterone, testosterone, DHEA, and cortisol.

But if your adrenals are constantly stressed, it can set off a painful autoimmune inflammatory response throughout your body. Your immunity and all your organs can be negatively impacted by the resulting high cortisol levels, which ultimately leads to degenerative disease.

Keep in mind that hypothyroidism and Hashimoto's are often misdiagnosed as adrenal fatigue because the symptoms are so similar. It can be difficult to interpret the tests for thyroid and adrenal problems, and many doctors simply do not believe in the connection except in the case of Addison's disease, an autoimmune disease in which the adrenals fail to produce enough cortisol, requiring lifelong cortisol replacement. Because many doctors do not believe in low thyroid function's connection to adrenal stress, fatigue, or insufficiency, it is *you* who must PUSH for your recovery!

Adrenal insufficiency symptoms include the following:

- Low blood pressure
- Low blood sugar
- Food and salt cravings
- Weakness
- Lack of libido
- Allergies
- Dark circles under the eyes
- Muscle and joint pain
- Dizziness
- Weakness
- Tendency to startle easily
- Lowered immune function
- Anxiety
- Depression
- Premature aging
- Poor sleep
- Dry skin
- Cystic breasts
- Lines of dark pigment in nails
- Difficulty recuperating from stresses, such as colds or jet lag
- No stamina for confrontation

Some of these symptoms are similar to those of low thyroid, which include the following:

- Cold hands and feet
- Fatigue and sluggishness
- Dry skin and scalp
- Thinning hair and/or hair loss
- Outer third of eyebrows thinning or missing
- Headaches and/or migraines
- Mental sluggishness
- Depression and lack of motivation
- Weight gain in spite of exercise and low-calorie diet
- Constipation or infrequent bowel movements
- No sweating

Remember! If you have hypothyroidism or Hashimoto's with the above adrenal symptoms and are placed on thyroid hormone alone, you may respond negatively. If you are not aware that you have an adrenal issue and begin treating your thyroid, the adrenal issue may surface and make the problem much worse rather than resolving it.

Once you are, in fact, diagnosed with thyroid disease—and again, most cases are autoimmune Hashimoto's thyroid disease—you must pay attention to supporting your adrenal glands. In order for your thyroid medication to work efficiently, your adrenals need support too. In the case of long-standing thyroid disease and the stress of it, along with stressful life events, the amount of stress overextends the capacity of your adrenal glands to compensate and recover. Once this capacity to cope and recover is exceeded, it is safe to assume that anyone with thyroid issues must support the health of the second most overlooked glands as well: the adrenals.

Who Suffers From Thyroid and Adrenal Issues?

The answer to this question is simply anyone who does not rest enough, play enough, or eat the right kinds of food enough. To go deeper, it is someone who drives herself too hard, is a perfectionist, or feels as if she is under pressure with no escape hatch. It is someone who has experienced chronic illness (undiagnosed thyroid disease fits the bill, by the way), who has experienced emotional trauma, or for whom physical injury set the stage for a thyroid-adrenal meltdown. The cost is untold frustration when it comes to the hours, months, and even years of unhappiness, poor health, loss of productivity, and lack of family interaction, a fulfilling love life, and creative ideas.

One thing to always remember, especially if your thyroid disease is autoimmune, is that whatever affects the thyroid will affect the adrenals, and whatever affects the adrenals will affect the thyroid. As your thyroid and adrenal health decline, you will find it increasingly difficult to handle any and all types of stress. You will also find yourself getting sick after stressful events, even if the events are a good kind of stress, such as the marriage of a child, the birth of a grandchild, or a wonderful trip.

What can you do if you feel this may be you? What if you are taking thyroid medication but still feel unwell? It could be that your adrenal glands need to be supported at the same time you are addressing your thyroid gland.

Again, it is very important to remember to support your adrenals while you are taking thyroid medication. The degree of adrenal involvement can vary. Support can come from natural supplements, or for a more severe case you may need hydrocortisone in a physiological dose (20 mg daily). Please note that if you have Hashimoto's disease, there may be a chance your adrenal issues are autoimmune as well. Have the health-care provider that has agreed to partner with you run a blood test for adrenal antibodies.

KNOW WHAT MOST DOCTORS DON'T

One clear indicator that adrenal problems are behind your situation is that you continue to have problems even after being prescribed proper amounts of thyroid hormone. I know this all too well because it happened to my daughters and me. I stated this before, but it is worth repeating: low adrenal gland function, meaning low cortisol, can actually cause your thyroid problem to be much worse than it would be otherwise.

You now know that if you have hypothyroidism, you need to be aware of your adrenal hormone levels, since many of the symptoms of low-functioning adrenals are the same as those of a low-functioning thyroid. I encourage you to be your own advocate, because even in this day and age, many doctors still dismiss adrenal problems except for cases of Addison's disease (extreme decreased adrenal function) or Cushing's syndrome (extreme increased adrenal function). It has been my personal experience that many doctors simply do not believe in anything in between.

In my opinion a single urine test, which most conventional doctors will prescribe, is not an accurate way to test true adrenal function. You have different levels of hormones in your urine at different times of the day. Therefore, it would be more effective to collect samples four or five different times of the day—morning, midmorning, afternoon, mid afternoon, and evening—to gather a more accurate snapshot of your daily adrenal function. The Adrenal Stress Index (ASI) test is the most accurate way to determine the degree of dysfunction when progress is being made.

Now that you are armed with this information, you may be tempted to self-treat your condition. But it is best to consult with a natural endocrine doctor or functional medicine physician. It takes a combination of factors to get you feeling well again. Simply going to the health store and buying adrenal or thyroid supplements is not enough. You need a well-versed endocrinologist, naturopath, or functional medicine doctor to evaluate you properly, thus saving you from doing years of guesswork on your own.

Low adrenal function is a difficult condition, and when it is accompanied by a thyroid issue, it can make you feel even worse. Believe me, I know this from personal experience. But the good news is that in most cases, people with low adrenal gland function can respond to a natural treatment protocol, or if necessary, physiological doses of cortisol. If you suspect you have adrenal issues—and if you have thyroid issues, you probably do—you should consult a functional medicine physician, an endocrinologist who is aware of how life-disrupting low adrenal output can be, or a naturopathic doctor. With the help of one of these doctors, there is an excellent chance that you can address both thyroid and adrenal issues simultaneously and regain your health.

The Risk of a Wrong Diagnosis

Before I was diagnosed with Hashimoto's thyroiditis, I had frequent panic attacks. I would hyperventilate on planes, while driving to the TV studio in Orlando, in grocery stores, while waiting in lines, and more, none of which I had ever done before. As time went on, I would nearly black out with tunnel vision and yell out to my family to call an ambulance because I thought I was having a cardiac event. I found myself asking for help more and more often, not knowing if I was soon going to take my last breath. These unfamiliar experiences were terrifying. I had consultations with cardiologists, allergists, and endocrinologists, and several hospital evaluations during those frightening years.

One time when I was driving on the busy I-4 freeway in Florida, I hyperventilated so badly that I blacked out at the wheel. By some miracle of God, I made it to the shoulder of the road and called 911.

Something was seriously wrong, and no doctor found it. Forty physicians in all dismissed my symptoms as stress and my busy career. I loved my career and did not feel any stress connected to it. It was exciting to help others, meet deadlines, travel, and be active doing what I felt God called me to do.

No, this was something else, which I tried in vain to explain to one doctor after another.

I made a life-changing move to Arizona, and my symptoms immediately became more intense. I have to admit the move was stressful, but it was very necessary! Once settled I began experiencing frequent infections. My joints and muscles ached. I was bone tired. I was having panic attacks daily. I could not go where I wanted or do what I needed to do because of the symptoms that baffled every doctor I consulted.

At the same time both of my daughters were getting much worse with their bewildering symptoms. My oldest daughter began having panic attacks, chronic infections, gut issues, and extreme fatigue. My youngest experienced daily migraines, insomnia, fatigue, and body pain. All three of us were stressed from not knowing what was causing us to not function as we once had. I can tell you that as a mother, it was unbelievably stressful to know that my children were sick and I was unable to help.

None of us knew our thyroids were being attacked by our immune systems and our adrenals were working overtime to pick up the slack. In the process our poor adrenals took a big hit. Now they were underfunctioning as well!

When your adrenals and thyroid aren't working, the impact on your day-to-day life and your ability to do the things you want or have to do can be devastating.

My daughters and I all had underlying adrenal issues that doctors dismissed as nothing when clearly we all were doing very badly after thyroid supplementation. My youngest daughter and I had severe issues with our adrenals after our thyroid cancers and resultant thyroidectomies. Our adrenal glands were producing very little cortisol. Because of this, we suffered for several years with dizziness, pain, swelling, a diagnosis of rheumatoid arthritis, insomnia, low blood sugar, weakness, and lowered immune function, just to name a few.

Since thyroid hormone medication can unmask very disturbing low adrenal output or low cortisol, the best thing to do in this case is to treat the patient with thyroid and adrenal support at the same time. This is very important!

Adrenal insufficiency is unpleasant and uncomfortable to say the least, especially when it is unmasked by taking thyroid hormone medication. I have experienced it, and so have my daughters. It is no fun. To make things even more difficult, your doctor may wrongly assume that your thyroid hormone medication is not right for you, or has even been a mistake! This is worrisome because precious time may be wasted while the patient only needed a little adrenal support to help the thyroid medication get into the tissues.

This happened to my daughters and me, and I don't want it to happen to you!

Something good can still come out of your symptoms, although they may be life disrupting and uncomfortable. They can point your physician in the right direction of having you gradually take thyroid and adrenal hormones together until you reach optimal levels of both. This careful attention and adjusting can be time consuming for both you and your doctor. It can be frustrating at first, so be sure to seek out a physician who will partner with you to see you through the demanding and sometimes frightening balancing process.

My two daughters were mostly housebound until the doctors listened to my plea to test our adrenal gland function. The results? We had numbers that were in the ditch and close to the markers for Addison's disease, a disease where your body does not make enough cortisol to keep you alive.

I am writing this book to arm you with the fact that your thyroid and adrenal glands are intricately connected. You must take care of both!

What I Wish I Knew Then

You are more likely to have a panic or anxiety attack if you have elevated thyroid antibodies. If you are suddenly experiencing panic attacks, it can be the first clue that you have an underlying autoimmune thyroid disease. Stress can trigger autoimmune thyroid issues by taxing and depleting your adrenal glands, which leads to anxiety and/or panic attacks.

If your adrenal fatigue is caught early, then in addition to optimal thyroid hormone treatment, adrenal glandular supplements, vitamin C, pantothenic acid, licorice, and chromium can help support your depleted, overworked adrenal glands. If your adrenal fatigue is severe, however, low-dose hydrocortisone given in appropriate doses can reverse your negative symptoms and dramatically improve your quality of life.

A special note to those of you who are already on thyroid medication: if you are experiencing panic attacks and/or high anxiety, you should definitely have your adrenal status checked. If your cortisol is low, you will need adrenal support. Also, your ability to convert T4 to active T3 needs to be assessed, because you may need a new thyroid medication. This is especially true if you are on a synthetic thyroid hormone replacement, such as Synthroid. You may need to make the big switch to a natural desiccated thyroid hormone, such as Armour or Nature-Throid, since they contain the thyroid hormones T4 and T3 along with T1 and T2. These formulations more closely match your body's own physiological levels. Panic can also be caused by imbalanced estrogen/progesterone levels. If you are in doubt, have all of these things measured.

The Impact of Stress

You must remember that low thyroid function is almost always secondary to some other condition, often adrenal stress.[1] The causes are many. In my case I have always lived a stress-filled life, beginning in childhood. I am an extreme type A personality, but thyroid and adrenal issues have downgraded me to a B-minus. A stressful life, blood sugar swings, food intolerances, chronic viruses, gut infections, and environmental toxins can all send your adrenals into overdrive, causing them to pump out cortisol. Adrenals on overdrive are dangerous and can result in autoimmunity.

Your thyroid is extremely dependent upon the health of

your adrenals. It is paramount for you to make sure you are doing all that you can to support their function. Failure to do so will simply make you feel wired, tired, and worse.

THE HOOKUP BETWEEN THE TWO

If you have hypothyroidism or autoimmune Hashimoto's disease, there is bound to be an adrenal component. How do you find out, and what tests are most accurate?

My daughters and I all had blood (serum) and twenty-four-hour urine tests done, as well as an ACTH test. All tests came back in the low normal range, indicating we were one or two points from an Addison's disease diagnosis. Conventional medicine goes by the blood work more than the patient's symptoms. I consulted naturopaths in Arizona, and all agreed to have an Adrenal Stress Index (ASI) test performed. This test is performed by Diagnos-Techs lab. This test is more sensitive and the most accurate. It helps to show how much cortisol your body is producing in a twenty-four-hour period and determines the state of your adrenal health.

There are seven stages to determine adrenal dysfunction according to the ASI test. Unfortunately my youngest daughter and I were already in stage seven by the time we received our diagnoses. Many people who fall into the stage seven range are housebound with no energy to live life normally. That is how serious my youngest daughter and I were. The *alarm reaction* is where your cortisol levels raise to help you adapt to increased stress levels. The *resistance stage* is when prolonged stress causes your body to "rob Peter to pay Paul," in terms of hormones. In this stage your body steals pregnenolone from cholesterol to make more cortisol. This will result in hormonal imbalances, because pregnenolone is needed to make your sex hormones. Typically you will see someone is this stage suffer from PMS and other hormonal issues related to the reproductive system, such as PCOS and infertility. Finally there is the *exhaustion stage*. It is this stage that my daughter and I wound up in. Our adrenal glands were exhausted and could not adapt to stress. Our adrenals were not able to make enough cortisol. We, in turn, did not have enough energy to do the many things in life that people take for granted.

My youngest daughter had all the signs of adrenal exhaustion, including all the symptoms of thyroid disease. I now know they go hand in hand. She was diagnosed at age thirteen with insulin resistance, anemia, metabolic syndrome, hormonal imbalance, and weight gain. She dealt with all of this before her Hashimoto's diagnosis years later. Without the knowledge that her adrenals needed supporting, she suffered for years. My oldest daughter and I suffered from panic attacks, shortness of breath, fatigue, and muscle stiffness. These were all signs of thyroid and adrenal issues. It was ten years later that the Hashimoto's diagnosis came, but that was only the beginning of our next ten-year battle to get well.

In order to drive this autoimmune thyroid disease into remission, we had to go deep into its many and varied causes. The adrenal glands needed intensive care. I spoke with John C. Lowe during these trying years. He was a brilliant educator on all things thyroid; he has since passed away. He told me to address those adrenal glands right away, and that our thyroid/autoimmune issues would not abate until the adrenals were addressed.

But why did all three of us have severe adrenal issues?

Adrenal stress impacts thyroid function. It is important to remember what I told you earlier about the way the gut, through gluten intolerance, inflammation, and leaky gut, can lead to the development of Hashimoto's. What leads to an unhealthy gut? Adrenal stress!

Adrenal stress can also be called adrenal fatigue, adrenal exhaustion, adrenal apathy, adrenal neurasthenia, subclinical hypoadrenia, or non-Addison's hypoadrenia. Millions of people in the United States and around the world are affected by symptoms that rob them of a productive life, and yet conventional medicine still fails to recognize adrenal fatigue as a distinct syndrome.[2]

Adrenal fatigue or exhaustion commonly occurs after periods of high or prolonged stress. It often occurs during or following *physically* stressful events such as acute or chronic infection, especially respiratory infections such as sinus infections, influenza, bronchitis, or pneumonia, with the main symptom being fatigue or lethargy that is not alleviated by sleep.[3] It can also happen after *emotionally* stressful events such as a painful divorce, job loss, or a death in the family, especially if all these things occur within months of each other, as they sometimes do.

What makes it so hard for others to understand is the fact that with adrenal fatigue, you may not have any outward signs of illness, yet you live with an overall feeling of unwellness. You may act normal on the outside, but inside you feel drained. Anyone who has lived with adrenal fatigue knows all too well how often they have to use caffeinated beverages, energy drinks, or foods to meet the challenges that each day brings.

Adrenal fatigue can wreak havoc on your life, changing you from a once-active member of society to someone who is withdrawn and depressed. In more serious cases the activity of the adrenal glands is so diminished that a person may be able to get out of bed for only a few hours a day. In addition, many people become homebound and may require a home health aide.

As adrenal function decreases, every organ and system of your body is more dramatically affected. Changes occur in your metabolism of carbohydrates, proteins, and fat; fluid and electrolyte balance; heart and cardiovascular system; and libido. In response your biochemical and cellular levels try to compensate for the decrease in adrenal hormones. Your body tries hard to make up for underfunctioning adrenal glands, but there is a price.[4]

What makes this all so complex is the fact these are the same symptoms of thyroid disease. The majority of people with these complaints are thrown into the category of "thyroid ill, so let's give her a pill." This was the case for my daughters and me. I know there are millions more out there who are not being optimally treated because many practitioners of conventional medicine refuse to look deeper and broader at the health of their patients' adrenal glands. Since the thyroid and adrenals work in tandem, it is imperative to support them both. I keep stressing this point because it will save you years of misery.

Go After It

What can you do right now? Be proactive in terms of your adrenal recovery. Every thyroid condition has an adrenal component. Start to support your body's batteries—the adrenals—now, whether you are currently seeking a thyroid diagnosis or are already being treated but your adrenals have been unsupported.

Here are two easy self-tests to see how well your adrenals are performing:

1. Postural Blood Pressure Test: To perform this first test, simply lie down and rest for five minutes. Then take your blood pressure.

When the five minutes are up, stand up and immediately take your blood pressure once more. If you notice that your blood pressure is lower after you stand up, it is a good indication that you probably have reduced adrenal gland function, which means your "batteries" need charging! The lower the blood pressure, the more severe the low adrenal function. The number on top of the blood pressure reading, otherwise known as the *systolic pressure*, is normally about ten points lower when you are lying down than when you are standing up. If you find that you have a difference of more than ten points, you should immediately begin following the suggestions I mentioned about recharging and supporting your weak adrenal glands.

2. Iris Contraction Test: For this next test simply sit in a darkened room in front of a mirror for about twenty seconds. Take a flashlight and shine it across your eye from the side of your face. Hold the light at eye level, but aim it toward your ear to avoid shining it directly into your eye. If you are dealing with poor adrenal function or are in a hypoadrenal state, your pupil will not be able to hold on to its contraction for more than twenty or thirty seconds. You may see your pupil "bounce" as it tries its very best to hold on to the contraction, but it will soon give out and remain dilated even though the flashlight is repeatedly shining around it. In persons with

> healthy adrenal function, the contraction normally holds and should last much longer.
>
> This test was first described by Dr. C. F. Arroyo in 1924 and measures the contraction of the iris in response to repeated exposure to dark light. His theory is that in those with weakened adrenal function, the iris will be unable to maintain its contraction for long. As a rule of thumb, the shorter the contraction time, the more severe your adrenal problem. This test has been used as a tool to detect hypoadrenia for many years by natural health practitioners and is deemed very accurate.[5]

In every case of adrenal recovery, you must focus on your diet. Some foods support adrenal function, while others create inflammation that taxes the adrenals even more. You must remove anything from your life that taxes your adrenals.

Know your enemies

We rely on many habits and substances—little comforts—to get us through each day, especially when suffering from constant fatigue. But this is when we need to be more vigilant. The following culprits can make adrenal fatigue even worse.

Stress

The number one enemy of your adrenal glands is stress. It taxes both adrenal and thyroid gland function because they work in tandem. Life automatically has a certain amount of stress, but most people quickly get into a state of stress overload. It isn't just the challenges we face; it is also how we react to those challenges. It is easy to magnify our difficulties to a crisis level. Our world is complicated, and we are submerged in worry over many things in our society today that human beings were never equipped to handle. All of this taxes the adrenals beyond their limits, and then our bodies declare an emergency in order to cope. We may not be able to change the world we live in, but we can learn to change how we perceive it and react to it.

Some very important techniques for handling stress include the identification of things in your life that are truly important and the establishment of boundaries to filter out those stressors that are not part of your basic priorities. Make a list of what is really important, and be tough on what makes the list. Write down what you really want to accomplish in life, and make note of how you can do it and what stands in your way. Do the same for your family members. Then make a list of people who are actually important in your life. It may seem cold, but then you need to make a list of people whose opinions don't really matter. This isn't about being mean; it is about doing what you have to do to regain your health. You must surrender your "disease to please." Some of these choices are hard but necessary. Once you have identified what should be inside the boundaries and what should be on the outside, make a plan to institute these boundaries and stick to them. It can be a huge adjustment and even a significant lifestyle change, but the health you will gain in the long run is well worth it.

Most of our life priorities are just collected from the circumstances we experience along the way. Few people deliberately design their life priorities in advance. We slowly develop into victims of circumstance rather than being in charge of our lives. The demands pile up, and the expectations can become overwhelming. As long as there isn't a plan, life will make one for you. Eventually you will have more than you can handle and your adrenals will be shot. This is where burnout comes from. If you continue to sacrifice your health just to keep juggling all the balls you have in the air, you will be on a sure pathway to a breakdown and serious health problems. Unless you take charge of it now, it will take charge of you later. One day you may find yourself in the grim situation where all the other demands of life stop in one moment and you will have just one priority—surviving.

Let me suggest some tips that will characterize the new you in a life where stress is managed properly:

- You have the ability to say no with no excuses.
- You don't need to be perfect; you are flexible and it's OK.
- You identify and participate in fun and relaxation with no guilt.
- You respect yourself and what you do without apology.
- You call in help when the tasks are too much—housekeepers, yard workers, etc.
- You pay more attention to your accomplishments than your failures.
- You think about your welfare and take care of yourself—put time and money into it.
- You exercise responsibly and let anger and frustration go through it.
- You don't take everything so seriously, because it isn't all that important.

- You laugh a lot more.
- You find supportive and cooperative friendships that don't drain you.
- You delegate responsibilities even if others can't do a task as well as you.
- You organize life events and calendars so you aren't worrying about them.

Notice that every tip started with the word *you*. Others are not in charge of your stress. *You* are. No one else can decide for you, unless you keep going and your decline in health takes over your life for you.

Sugar

The next big enemy of your adrenal health is sugar. When the adrenal glands are exhausted, they can't produce enough adrenaline to keep your energy levels normal. They begin to crave a source of quick energy for a boost, and your body knows where to find it. Glucose is the substance, and the body can quickly get it from sugar. You will want candy, sodas, pastries, breads, muffins, rolls, cakes, pies, and any of the multitude of drinks and processed food products on the market that contain sugar, high-fructose corn syrup, and other sweeteners. You must be careful because things labeled natural are not necessarily low sugar. My all-time favorite sweetener is Stevia. It is an herb from South America that is two hundred times sweeter than sugar and has zero calories. It gives a wonderful sweetness to my decaf coffee and iced tea or other foods.

Caffeine

Along with stress and sugar, the next enemy is caffeine. It will provide the body with a fast energy boost when the adrenals fall short. There are obvious sources that must be replaced by decaffeinated substitutes, but you also need to become an avid label reader because food manufacturers love to hide caffeine in the most unlikely places. Like sugar, caffeine is addictive, and all the more so when you need the energy it supplies. Food and drink manufacturers know this and depend on the profits they can gain when people become addicted to their products. Your adrenals deserve better! You don't want to get on the cycle of merely swapping one problem for another. It's time to become your body's energy manager. Another problem with caffeine is the imbalance it brings to your sleep. It makes it hard to go to sleep at night and hard to wake up in the morning. Healing the adrenals requires good sleep, and caffeine will work against every effort you make to get your body in sync.

Leaky gut and gluten

Most people with adrenal problems suffer with other energy-robbing issues as well. One key problem is leaky gut syndrome, which is a culprit in food allergies, chronic systemic and gastrointestinal inflammation, and autoimmunity. It is interesting to realize that most of these problems can be traced back to another one of your enemies—wheat gluten. Gluten is in so much of the food we buy and eat, and anyone with an allergy or sensitivity to it will feel the effects soon after they eat it. In addition to causing you to feel bad, it can also be a catalyst in a cascade of other suspected diseases. Gluten is strongly implicated in Hashimoto's disease. I recommend that you avoid not only wheat gluten but also *all* grains and legumes, since they can also react upon your thyroid in a negative way.

Food supply

The mystery of the modern food supply is filled with things that are more often bad for you than good. Laboratories are busy filling our processed foods with new chemicals and nutritional sources that have had their DNA tampered with. In a corporate effort to make everything cheaper and faster, we have lost the importance of making it better. Why are there so many ads on TV for digestion and heartburn remedies now? These test tube foods are harder to digest, and they tax your body, sleep, and adrenals. It is so common now to see foods that are filled with hydrogenated oils, and those soybean, canola, and corn oils are hard to digest. It is time to select good, healthier fats such as coconut oil, olive oil, and organic butter, and to cook your own healthy foods as much as possible.

Lack of sleep

The importance of sleep can't be overstated. Stop and rest when you feel tired. Take naps. Get eight to ten hours of sleep every night, and go to bed before 10:00 p.m. When you are on a consistent sleep cycle and avoid staying up too late, your adrenals will have a much better chance to recover.

Boost your adrenals

The following can help give your adrenals the boost they need:

- Pantothenic acid, a B vitamin known as the antistress vitamin
- B-complex vitamins
- Vitamin C
- Ashwagandha

- Astragalus
- Adrenal complex glandular supplement
- Zinc
- Selenium

If your adrenal glands do not bounce back with these recommendations, the next step to consider is the use of bioidentical hormones. This can be especially true if you are taking thyroid medication and not feeling better. Many people with thyroid issues also have sluggish adrenals, which makes it hard for the body to utilize thyroid medication efficiently. Blood tests can help to determine where hormonal deficiencies lie.

For severe adrenal fatigue appropriate doses of cortisol (hydrocortisone) are often needed. My daughters and I had stage 7 adrenal fatigue long before our Hashimoto's and papillary thyroid cancer diagnoses. My youngest daughter was mostly housebound but managed to get out now and then. Hydrocortisone was the answer for us, along with finding the right thyroid medication.

Bioidentical cortisol can also be prescribed for severe adrenal fatigue. It has been used for decades to treat adrenal insufficiency and Addison's disease. Extensive research by William McK. Jefferies, which can be found in his book *Safe Uses of Cortisol*, shows that hydrocortisone, in doses of 5 mg four times daily, can bring life back into the adrenal glands and to the patient. In addition, hydrocortisone can help manage autoimmune disorders such as Hashimoto's by giving the body what it needs to quiet widespread inflammation and to help the body utilize thyroid hormone medication.[6]

The aim of adrenal fatigue treatment is to get the

adrenals working again. Because of this it's important to know that there are other hormone deficiencies that occur with adrenal exhaustion. Every six months, to ensure that my hormonal levels are optimal, I have the following tests performed by a health-care provider who is well versed in bioidentical hormone replacement.

1. DHEA: It is very common for people who suffer from low adrenal function to have low levels of DHEA, which is an important precursor to testosterone and other sex hormones. Many physicians who are well versed in bioidentical hormone replacement therapy believe that saliva testing is the most reliable way to determine the optimal replacement dose of DHEA. If DHEA is replenished and brought back to optimal levels, it can lead to a return of sex drive and energy as well as other general markers of vitality, such as a feeling of well-being that is often lost or forgotten during adrenal fatigue.

   Something to take note of here is that DHEA replacement should always be accompanied by regular testing because it can convert easily into testosterone. Women should take special note of this, as it can lead to masculinization side effects such as hirsutism, or excessive and abnormal hair growth. Starting with a small dose is recommended.

2. Pregnenolone: This is known as the grandmother of all hormones. It can convert to whatever hormone is needed (sex or stress

hormones) in the correct amounts. If you have reduced levels of sex hormones or stress hormones, a pregnenolone supplement might improve your symptoms.

Pregnenolone is often taken in oral capsule form. For those persons in stage 3 or 4 of adrenal fatigue, starting with a small dose is advisable. Work with your health-care provider concerning all hormone replacement dosing.

3. Testosterone: It is well known that men need testosterone. But did you know that women need it too? While it is true that women only produce a fraction of the amount needed by men, it is still an important player when it comes to a woman's vitality and improving things like libido, endurance, and mood. If you are suffering from adrenal fatigue, talk to your doctor about the benefits of restoring your testosterone to optimal levels.

   I can personally attest to this, as I spent the first half of my life receiving testosterone subcutaneous pellets implanted into my hip every six months to help my adrenals function normally, and to ease the burden placed upon them by my yet-to-be-diagnosed thyroid disease. Just like DHEA, too much testosterone can cause masculinization such as hirsutism (unwanted excess hair growth), so testing for your ideal dose is key.

4. Estrogen: If you are a woman who is experiencing adrenal fatigue, bioidentical estrogen

replacement therapy can make a world of difference. Adrenal fatigue can create a deficiency of all of your hormones, including estrogen. But estrogen deficiency typically happens later in the condition's progression. Be sure to work with a health-care professional who is well versed in bioidentical hormone replacement to ensure that you are getting the right dose, specially tailored to your needs.

5. Progesterone: Progesterone is known as the hormone of well-being, and when it starts to drop, your well-being goes right out the window! Progesterone will drop before your estrogen levels change, usually around perimenopause during the mid to late thirties for women, and this can cause weight gain, irritability, and lower energy levels. It is interesting to note here that progesterone actually facilitates thyroid function, and women with low thyroid and/or adrenal function traditionally have low progesterone levels. For women who are experiencing adrenal fatigue, the "pregnenolone steal" that occurs in a desperate attempt to keep things running smoothly from a hormonal perspective results in your progesterone levels plummeting even lower. This is when progesterone replacement can come to your rescue, so to speak, and pull you back from the brink of despair. Again, work with a health-care provider who is well trained in bioidentical hormone replacement therapy.

Give it time

You must be patient, because you essentially *are* a "patient." Recovery from adrenal fatigue can take time. Remember that it took a long time—months or even years—to exhaust your precious adrenals, so it makes sense that it will also take time to build up their strength again. To experience full adrenal recovery, you must implement all of the suggestions you have read as closely as possible. The following is a guide to the recovery time frame you can expect:

- Six to nine months for minor adrenal fatigue
- Twelve to eighteen months for moderate fatigue
- Up to twenty-four months for severe adrenal fatigue

It is important to remember that making solid changes to your diet and lifestyle is the best way to see lasting results. Like I have always said, "Take care of your adrenal glands, and they will take care of you!"

Implement these adrenal support tips while you are waiting for diagnosis, or if you are already diagnosed and trying to get proper treatment. Use these tips if you are treated optimally and are feeling well. Remember, the thyroid and adrenals are *sympatico*—they need each other to be functioning at full capacity.

Adrenal fatigue is more prevalent than you can imagine. Noted author and expert in all things adrenal James L. Wilson, ND, DC, PhD, estimates that around 80 percent of people worldwide suffer from this malady. He believes that at some point in their lives, most people are going to struggle with adrenal fatigue either as a short-term or chronic problem.[7] My daughters and I have suffered from adrenal fatigue to the point of nearly developing acute adrenal insufficiency or Addison's disease, meaning we weren't producing enough cortisol to keep us functioning. At the time none of us knew (and I am the expert here) that our poorly functioning thyroids were taxing our adrenal glands to near collapse!

Take care of your adrenals, and they will take care of you!

> If you are too debilitated to look things up online, get Dr. Janet's books. Dr. Janet helped pull me through in 2006. Her adrenal support suggestions were a lifeline. Knowing there was a woman out there who truly knew what I was going through and was willing to help me out of the "thyroid ditch" was heaven sent.
>
> God bless you, Dr. Janet!
>
> With utmost respect,
> Catherine Granton

Chapter 6

THE THYROID AND THE HEART

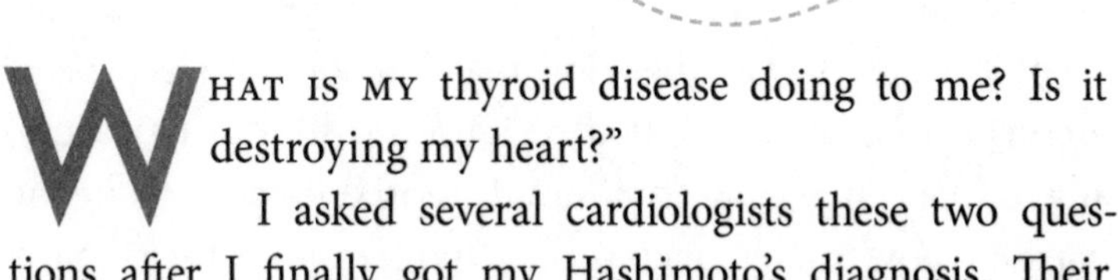

"WHAT IS MY thyroid disease doing to me? Is it destroying my heart?"

I asked several cardiologists these two questions after I finally got my Hashimoto's diagnosis. Their answer was, "It's just stress." My frightening symptoms were:

- High blood pressure
- Low blood pressure
- Slow/weak pulse (under 60 bpm)
- Fast pulse (over 90 bpm at rest)
- Arrhythmia
- Skipped beats
- Heart palpitations
- Chest pain
- Air hunger/shortness of breath
- High cholesterol
- High triglycerides
- High LDL ("bad") cholesterol
- Mitral valve prolapse
- High C-reactive protein

- Fibrillation
- Poor circulation

In addition, all my female relatives have high cholesterol and are on statin drugs. I have recently found out that my relatives have been diagnosed with Hashimoto's disease too. All of it makes me wonder: How many people who have been prescribed statins and blood pressure medications are actually in fact suffering from undiagnosed hypothyroidism? Further, how many diagnosed hypothyroid patients have been poorly managing their condition and have been placed on statins and blood pressure medications when all that is needed is a thyroid medication change or dosage increase?

I have flashbacks of the many times I sat in my cardiologist's office trying to find out why my cholesterol was extremely high, my heart rate was irregular, and I was so short of breath that I experienced panic attacks. As I sat in the waiting room, I looked at the patients sitting and waiting for yet another exam and medication to control their symptoms. Considering what I have learned and experienced firsthand, I wonder just how many of those patients in that waiting room were actually yet-to-be-diagnosed or undertreated hypothyroid sufferers. (I was!) In a perfect world I believe that heart patients should be treated for thyroid issues *before* medications are prescribed or heart surgery is performed. My family members were not tested or treated for thyroid issues, which leaves me to wonder if our loved ones who have died of heart attacks, strokes, or other heart disease complications could have fared better and had a longer and better quality of life here on Earth *if* they'd had their thyroid levels measured and treated.

I am on thyroid replacement hormones now, and am happy to tell you that for the first time in my life my cholesterol is normal, and my shortness of breath that plagued me for twenty years is gone! I believe that my experience can somehow heal my family's past, present, and certainly the future generations by having this culprit (thyroid disease) unearthed and exposed, never to follow our family line for generations again.

Then there is the article that appeared in 2007 in *Circulation*, a scientific journal published for the American Heart Association, titled "Cardiovascular Involvement in General Medical Conditions: Thyroid Disease and the Heart." It said:

> The cardiovascular signs and symptoms of thyroid disease are some of the most profound and clinically relevant findings that accompany both hyperthyroidism and hypothyroidism. On the basis of the understanding of the cellular mechanisms of thyroid hormone action on the heart and cardiovascular system, it is possible to explain the changes in cardiac output, cardiac contractility, blood pressure, vascular resistance, and rhythm disturbances that result from thyroid dysfunction. The importance of the recognition of the effects of thyroid disease on the heart also derives from the observation that restoration of normal thyroid function most often reverses the abnormal cardiovascular hemodynamics.[1]

And according to the Thyroid Federation International:

> The heart is a major target of thyroid hormones. Any change in thyroid hormone levels will be responded to by the heart.
>
> Too little thyroid hormone is a consequence of an underactive thyroid (hypothyroidism):
>
> [It] causes your heart to beat too slowly or

> irregularly, to flutter with missing or additional beats. As a consequence bradycardia may develop; this form of arrhythmia leaves your organs and tissues without enough oxygen and nutrients. Severe bradycardia can result in cardiac arrest. [It] causes your blood pressure to change. Over time, high blood pressure will develop with the consequence of developing atherosclerosis, a risk for heart attack and stroke. [It] causes your cholesterol in the blood to rise and calcification, so called plaque, to develop in your arteries and makes them stiff. All these effects increase the risk for heart attack, heart failure and atherosclerosis.[2]

According to the World Heart Federation, heart disease ranks as the number one killer of women worldwide.[3]

The Thyroid Federation International estimates that up to 300 million people worldwide have thyroid dysfunction, and the majority of them are women. Remember, more than half of them are likely to be unaware of their condition.[4]

It makes you wonder: Is heart disease the real killer of women? Or is it really undiagnosed or undertreated thyroid disease?

Let's get scientific.

Cardiac Symptoms of Hypothyroidism—Getting to the Heart of the Matter

When you have thyroid disease, whether it be hypothyroidism, hyperthyroidism, Graves' disease, or Hashimoto's disease, you will most likely deal with cardiac symptoms that serve as a "tip off" long before your actual diagnosis. This is especially true if you already have an underlying heart issue such as mitral valve prolapse, other heart valve issues, or congestive heart failure. It is common to have the following cardiac symptoms associated with hypothyroidism, and Hashimoto's thyroiditis in particular:

Shortness of breath or air hunger

Dyspnea, or shortness of breath, in hypothyroidism is often caused by weakness in the skeletal muscles, but if you already have existing heart disease, the shortness of breath may be due to worsening of your preexisting heart condition. What's more, many people report having panic attacks due to this troubling symptom. My oldest daughter and I found this to be one of the worst symptoms we had to endure before our diagnoses of Hashimoto's.

Slow heart rate

Thyroid hormone regulates your heart rate (pulse). Bradycardia—a pulse that is 10–20 beats per minute slower than normal—is typical in hypothyroidism, and so is an increased tendency for premature heartbeats. Hypothyroidism may cause atrial fibrillation.

Hypertension

Many people may guess that since hypothyroidism slows down the metabolism, it might also cause low blood pressure. It did for my daughters and me. Our blood pressure readings were always very low, but it was mostly due to our extremely taxed adrenal glands. Our poor adrenal function threw our fluid balance out of whack, and it took years for us to know that electrolyte replacement would be our salvation. For many people, however, the opposite is true, as the arteries are stiffer in hypothyroid patients. That causes blood pressure to rise, which can make heart failure much worse, or can actually cause heart failure in people who did not have a preexisting case.

Heart failure is a major cause of death in the United

States and Europe. You should know that hypothyroidism can make even well-managed heart failure worse. What's more, hypothyroidism can contribute to heart failure in patients with mild underlying heart disease, especially if their thyroid disease is poorly managed.

Edema or swelling

Swelling, particularly of the extremities, also known as edema, can be a clear sign that heart failure is worsening. Thyroid patients may experience a specific type of edema called myxedema, which can contribute to coronary artery disease (CAD). What I know now is that a reduction in thyroid hormone production can cause an increase in LDL cholesterol (bad cholesterol) and in C-reactive protein (CRP). My levels of both LDL and CRP were sky-high, and not one doctor I consulted made the connection! This is vital for you to know because these clues that point to hypothyroidism can also accelerate or contribute to any underlying coronary artery disease.

As I have stated, hypothyroidism is often an insidious condition. It most often has a very slow onset, and its symptoms can be subtle. It is important to note that especially in older people, hypothyroidism can occur without the typical textbook symptoms that doctors usually expect. You must learn to be a thyroid detective, so to speak, looking for clues that point to this butterfly-shaped gland in your neck that can destroy your quality of life and make it a complete wreck. I believe that hypothyroidism is a silent epidemic that is more frequent than many doctors realize. So if you have any of these symptoms you have read about thus far and your doctor does not have a convincing explanation for them, especially if you already have heart disease of any type, PUSH! Ask your doctor to measure your thyroid hormone levels (TSH, TG, and TgAb). You just may save your own life!

Hyperthyroidism and the Heart—When the Pitter-Patter Matters!

I have not focused on the condition opposite hypothyroidism, hyperthyroidism, but it is important to discuss because it can be detrimental to the heart. This condition is aptly named because it will truly make you hyper. For that reason, it is much easier to recognize and diagnose.

When your body produces too much thyroid hormone, as in hyperthyroidism, your heart works overtime because having too much thyroid hormone increases the contraction and force of your heart muscle. This in turn increases your heart's demand for oxygen. But what most people find most worrisome is the resultant increase in heartbeat, a heart rhythm disorder called atrial fibrillation. With hyperthyroidism, the heart rate is often rapid even at rest, which can be the most frightening symptom by far![5]

This fast heart rate, otherwise known as tachycardia and palpitations, is the "calling card" of hyperthyroidism. It can occur when you're at rest or with mild exertion. When you visit a cardiologist because of an increased heart rate or "palps," be sure to ask him to consider hyperthyroidism, complete with blood tests, before he possibly makes a hasty diagnosis of inappropriate sinus tachycardia. It can happen!

Hyperthyroidism can cause a host of other cardiac symptoms, such as arrhythmia and premature beats. *Always* ask about a possible thyroid connection!

As with hypothyroidism, hyperthyroidism can be present without classic textbook symptoms, and it can be insidious. If you have any of these cardiac symptoms, please have your thyroid hormone levels checked!

- Dyspnea: Hyperthyroidism can be accompanied by dyspnea (shortness of breath) with even mild exertion. Muscle weakness or progressing heart failure created by hyperthyroidism can be the underlying cause of dyspnea.
- Heart failure: It is rare, but hyperthyroidism can cause heart failure. The difficult issue with hyperthyroidism is that if you have preexisting heart disease, worsening of your condition is very common and difficult to treat.
- Angina: What's more, in hyperthyroid patients with existing coronary artery disease, there is often a progression of their disease, including chest pain (angina) or even the most dreaded of all cardiac events: a heart attack.

WHEN THYROID LEVELS DROP, LIPIDS LEAP!

Most of you know that poor diet is the most common cause of high cholesterol, but I am certain that not too many of you know that the second-leading cause is hypothyroidism. My cholesterol was 357 at seventeen years old! How I wish someone would have made the connection back then. My life would have been much different. What I did not know then was that my thyroid hormone levels dropped, which made my liver take a hit. It no longer functioned optimally and began to produce excess cholesterol, fatty acids, and triglycerides. This increased my risk for atherosclerosis in the future, and ultimately heart disease.

It is good to know that some thyroid experts and astute cardiologists finally realize that there is a real relationship between hypothyroidism and chronically "wonky" lipid levels, namely elevated LDL (bad cholesterol), reduced HDL (good cholesterol), and elevated triglycerides. Even with my continually high cholesterol numbers and lipid levels, not one cardiologist suggested that my thyroid could be behind the extremely high and potentially dangerous readings.

I wonder just how many people, especially women, are currently taking statin medications, depleting their bodies of CoQ_{10}, to try to force their cholesterol down to acceptable levels, when addressing their underlying thyroid issue could make a huge difference not only in their cardiovascular health, but in every aspect of their lives.[6]

Leave It to the Italians!

Thyroid hormone replacement worked for me. My cholesterol and lipid levels are within acceptable levels for the first time in my life! And now there is a study to support it. An Italian research group selected a group of thyroid patients with elevated lipid levels. After six months of T4 thyroid medication, which created stable, normal T4 levels, the patients had a dramatic decrease in serum total cholesterol and LDL levels (unlike the patients placed on a placebo, who had not improved at all).[7] So the good news here is that T4 therapy can reduce LDL levels and thereby reduce the risk of atherosclerosis and heart disease![8]

Put Out That Cigarette!

Something you should consider: another study found that smoking can contribute to high cholesterol and lipid levels in women with subclinical hypothyroidism. So smoking increases the cardiovascular consequences of this disease.[9]

THYROID HORMONES—MORE GOOD NEWS!

Another exciting discovery from the Italians' research is that treating people who have subclinical hypothyroidism with thyroid hormones can prevent the progression to true hypothyroidism! What's more, the proper treatment can alleviate the myriad of annoying and life-disrupting symptoms of thyroid deficiency. And even better news is that it appears that the subclinical thyroid issue is reversible in at least 25 percent of patients! The most wonderful discovery for us all is that since many of the symptoms are associated with the aging process, alleviating them with the proper dose of thyroid hormone may make a person feel younger and vital again—and let's not forget all of the protective benefits your dear heart receives![10] *Grazie* to the Italians!

BEFORE STATINS, THINK THYROID!

Now you know that low thyroid hormone levels can contribute to a high risk of heart disease. If you have high cholesterol, before agreeing to take statin medications that have potentially dangerous side effects, have your thyroid and thyroid antibodies checked. By decreasing the levels of LDL (bad cholesterol) with optimal doses of thyroid medication, you may reduce the risk for atherosclerosis and heart disease.

My case: My cholesterol was dangerously high for most of my life. My total cholesterol reading at age seventeen was 357, and no matter what I tried, it remained over 300 for most of my life. Not one doctor suggested that it might be due to thyroid disease. Once my antibodies were checked at age fifty and I was found to have Hashimoto's thyroiditis, I started taking Nature-Throid and eliminated all grains from my diet, and I am happy to report that my cholesterol number has dropped almost one hundred points!

Chapter 7

THE THYROID AND BLOOD SUGAR

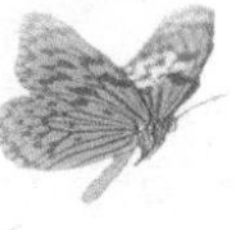

MY DAUGHTER SUFFERED from fainting spells due to low blood sugar, or hypoglycemia, before she got her thyroid diagnosis. It took years for doctors to discover this, as the simple blood tests they ran did not indicate there was an issue. It wasn't until they did a fasting glucose test that they discovered she had insulin resistance/metabolic syndrome—another tip-off that her thyroid was in trouble that was missed.

They were looking at a tree and missing the forest! Her entire endocrine system was a mess, and no doctor would hear my concerns about how it all was connected. I told them over and over that they needed to find the root cause—that is how I had always helped my clients—but this idea was foreign to them. I cannot put into words the frustration this journey brought to my daughter and me.

They're More Connected Than You Think

The American Thyroid Association estimates that 20 million Americans suffer from some form of thyroid disease, and up to 60 percent of them go undiagnosed.[1] What's more, women are five to eight times more likely to have thyroid issues than men.[2] Again, my daughters and I were three of them.

Thyroid disease can greatly affect your body's ability to handle blood sugar. It decreases the rate of glucose absorption in your gut, slows the rate of glucose uptake by your cells, and slows the clearance of insulin from your blood. In other words, thyroid disease s-l-o-w-s everything in your body, right down to the cellular level.

When this happens it is clinically known as hypoglycemia. But when you have hypothyroidism, your cells are resistant to glucose. This means that even when you have normal levels of glucose in your blood, you'll have the symptoms of hypoglycemia, such as fatigue, headache, hunger, irritability, dizziness, and more. My youngest daughter suffered terribly with these symptoms until her blood sugar issues were diagnosed and addressed. She had developed "insulin resistance" at a young age from a yet-to-be diagnosed thyroid condition, and not one doctor recognized it. It's hard to imagine, but again, it *can* happen!

When cells don't get enough glucose, the adrenal glands release cortisol to compensate. This cortisol release increases glucose, but it also sends a signal that a chronic stress response is underway, which in turn suppresses the function of the thyroid.

You may have heard of metabolic syndrome or know someone who suffers from it. This disorder is a combination of metabolic risk factors that happen at the same time and might seem to be unrelated, but they actually have the same cause in common—chronic hyperglycemia, or high blood sugar. The indicators are obesity, primarily in the abdominal area; insulin resistance; high blood pressure; high cholesterol; high triglycerides; frequent formation of blood clots; and inflammation that is not related to other issues.

Thirty-five percent of the US population lives with metabolic syndrome or insulin resistance. Insulin resistance is more common and is seen in nearly 105 million people in this country. The more complicated condition, metabolic syndrome, affects the lives of nearly 50 million.[3] Both of these conditions are associated with heart disease and diabetes, which are at the top of the list of causes of death in our society.[4] My youngest daughter is unfortunately a victim of thyroid disease, metabolic syndrome, insulin resistance, and papillary thyroid cancer.

The high parallel rates of both thyroid dysfunction and metabolic syndrome leads to suspicion that the two diseases are linked, and it is now confirmed! Research indicates that incidences of thyroid disorders are high in diabetics, and those with thyroid disorders are much more likely to experience metabolic syndrome and obesity. A healthy thyroid is the key to maintaining normal blood sugar levels, while it is also true that holding blood sugar levels in the normal range is vital to having a healthy thyroid.[5]

Eating excess carbohydrates forces the pancreas to secrete high levels of insulin to transfer the glucose in the blood into the cells, where that glucose can be used to create energy. This repeated, ongoing process becomes a condition called chronic hyperglycemia. As it progresses, the cells become resistant to insulin, so the pancreas creates more and more insulin in its attempt to manage the high glucose levels. As this situation worsens, it becomes what is called insulin resistance.

The high levels of insulin released in order to balance excess glucose are dangerous to other parts of the body, especially the thyroid gland. Insulin resistance is marked by continual surges of insulin that progressively destroy the thyroid gland, a process that is accelerated in those with autoimmune thyroid disease, or Hashimoto's. The result of this attack on the thyroid gland is the reduction of thyroid hormone production.

Just as high blood sugar can threaten your thyroid, low

blood sugar can be just as problematic. Long-standing hypoglycemia can cause coma, seizures, and death. Thankfully your body can detect low blood sugar. When blood sugar levels drop below normal, the adrenal glands answer the alarm and produce additional cortisol. This reaction creates another situation: now cortisol is ordering the liver to release more glucose, which will raise the blood sugar—but what is it doing to your thyroid gland in the process?

When the adrenal glands are called to action, cortisol is the hormone they produce. While it will effectively direct the correction of the low blood sugar event, cortisol is also a nervous system hormone that has a major role in the fight or flight mechanism. Its job is to help us react to an emergency by increasing the heartbeat and lung activity to produce greater blood flow to the skeletal muscles that are being called into action. When no emergency exists, cortisol supports other functions such as regulating the flow of glucose to the brain, supporting tissue repair, and modulating body functions that are not involved in a crisis, such as digestion, reproduction, and growth.

When cortisol is released too frequently, as is the case for hypoglycemics, it has an adverse effect on the pituitary gland. Once this reaction suppresses pituitary function, the imbalance then impacts the thyroid, causing it to malfunction as well.

In a cascade of one imbalance creating a myriad of others, both hyperglycemia and hypoglycemia disrupt many healthy and essential functions. These abnormal chemical reactions cause inflammation in the gut, lungs, and brain. They send hormones out of balance and deplete the adrenal glands. The conditions they create interfere with metabolism and detoxification, and can even lead to polycystic ovary syndrome. Since the thyroid gland is involved in all of these systems, the overload wears the thyroid down and reduces its ability to manage all of the other glands of the body. It's clear that your thyroid doesn't stand a chance when you have blood sugar issues.

You may now be seeing the tug of war that takes place between blood sugar issues and thyroid disease. It might appear confusing that both high and low blood sugar can be detrimental to your thyroid. It may be even more confusing that a thyroid problem can be causing hyperglycemia or hypoglycemia. This is the vicious circle your doctor must decode in order to treat you. It's also easy to see how your doctor could get confused about which issue is the underlying culprit.

As a starting point there is one approach that can address many of these questions: test to find out if you have blood sugar abnormalities, and then use self-monitoring to try to keep your blood sugar in the proper range. You can get the measurements you need by buying a simple blood glucose meter at a pharmacy and learning how to regularly perform self-tests. Keep a daily journal of your results and observe the trends. The readings will reveal important truth in your quest for answers.

The first test you need to become familiar with is the fasting glucose test. Your blood sugar is measured in the morning before you have anything to eat or drink. The number should be between 75 and 95, which stands for 75 to 95 mg/dL. If you consistently measure above 95, it is a warning sign that you may be headed for diabetes in the future.

The next test is called the postprandial blood glucose test. This measurement is performed one to two hours after a meal, and the number should decrease with time after eating. The number should be 120 mg/dL or less. Two hours after a meal, it is common for this number to have dropped to less than 100 mg/dL.

If you are hypoglycemic, meaning that your blood sugar tends to get too low, your goal is to keep your blood glucose above 75 mg/dL all day. The ideal way to do this is to eat a low-to-moderate-carbohydrate diet so you don't create any glucose spikes. When your glucose goes too high, it will ultimately come back down too low. Keeping your energy even with small, frequent meals is the pattern that will work best.

If you are hyperglycemic, meaning that your blood sugar gets too high, it is important that you design your diet and lifestyle to hold your postprandial glucose measurement below 120 mg/dL two hours after each of your meals. The only way to accomplish this is to restrict carbohydrates. How restrictive you need to be depends on the measurements you achieve. Be as strict as it takes to achieve the numbers you should produce.

In addition to this testing and self-monitoring, you must also have your thyroid properly checked and treated with supplemental hormones if needed. Since blood sugar problems and thyroid disorders influence each other, it is crucial to deal with both in order to effectively stabilize the overall situation effectively.

The good news here is that by getting your thyroid disease diagnosed and treated adequately (and changing your diet to low carb and gluten and grain free, if you have autoimmune thyroid disease), you will be on your way to regaining your health.

Is It Affecting You?

Are you wondering if your blood sugar handling ability is impaired? Here are some of the key symptoms of blood sugar imbalance:

Symptoms of hypoglycemia (low blood sugar)

- Having blurred vision
- Feeling light-headed if meals are missed
- Needing coffee to give you energy
- Being irritable if a meal is missed
- Feeling shaky or jittery
- Having trouble thinking, concentrating, and remembering things
- Craving sweets to feel better

Symptoms of insulin resistance

- Fatigue
- Morning nausea
- Your waist is equal to or larger than your hips
- Difficulty losing weight
- Frequent urination
- Always hungry
- Feeling tired after meals
- Feeling the need to have sweets after meals
- Aches and pains throughout your body

IT'S IN THE DIET

What can you do right now? If you can relate to these symptoms, you must change your diet right away. Do the following:

- Never skip breakfast. Have a low-carb, high-protein and high-fats breakfast. If you have nausea in the morning, a good breakfast with ample protein will help to quell it.
- Eat a small protein snack every two or three hours. Turkey, chicken, cheese, a hard-boiled egg, and some nuts are good examples.
- Limit all grains, as they are carbohydrates.
- Avoid stimulants like coffee and iced tea. Green tea is permissible. Iced tea and coffee tax your already weakened adrenals, which will in turn affect your thyroid health.
- Don't have sweets before bed. This will cause your blood sugar to crash overnight, causing poor sleep quality as your adrenals rally to help balance your system until your next meal, which is hours away. If you do eat sweets or carbs, make sure you balance it with a protein. The protein will help to slow down the rate at which the glucose is absorbed into your bloodstream.

You will find that cutting carbs or eating low carbs and high protein may even help you lose that weight that has been impossible to lose. It is all about endocrine balance. Balancing your blood sugar will help your thyroid condition. A diet full of sugar and starches will cause blood sugar swings that make it harder to heal your condition. Protein is slow, even-burning fuel that will keep your system on an even keel. The harder your body has to work to manage blood spikes and crashes, the less it can begin to normalize your thyroid/adrenal function.

In the case of autoimmune thyroid disease, you should know that sugars and starches aggravate autoimmunity. Eating a diet of lean protein, vegetables, small amounts of fruit, and no grains (especially gluten!) can help calm the autoimmune attack, keep your blood sugar balanced, and help you to lose weight.

I Cannot "Sugarcoat" It

Before my daughters and I were diagnosed with all of these interconnected endocrine conditions, the symptoms that caused so much angst were overlooked when I brought them to a physician's attention. My youngest daughter needed cola and food every two hours or so, which I tried to control, but being from an Italian family, I had people working against my efforts to curtail her eating. After all, food is everything when you're Italian!

As my youngest reached puberty, she began to really decline in terms of her health—always sick, always hungry, and always needing sugar or caffeine to keep going. It was more than "stress eating," and I knew it. But I yielded to her doctor when he said, "You worry too much. She just needs a hobby to take her mind off of food."

It wasn't until she began fainting and taking several trips to the hospital that she was given a three-hour glucose tolerance test. The test showed that she definitely had functional hypoglycemia, which meant that three hours after ingesting sugars, starches, or carbohydrates, her blood sugar crashed.

That is why she was fainting when she came home from school—it was about three hours after lunch!

At that time no one suspected that her immune system was attacking her thyroid and was at the root of her distress. She was given the drug Metformin to help with her blood sugar peaks and valleys. It did help, but not completely. She felt unwell every day with migraines, dizzy spells, fatigue, weight gain, cold extremities, and body aches. Her doctor said, "You see, Mama, at least she isn't fainting anymore."

This all occurred when she became a teenager. Her Hashimoto's thyroid disease was not diagnosed until she was twenty-four. That's ten long years of symptoms mounting up with no answers. Her life came to a standstill. It was hard for her, and it was very hard for me to see my girl suffer more and more with each passing year.

It was only when I received my Hashimoto's diagnosis that I pushed to have my girls tested. We all had autoimmune thyroid disease of a long-standing nature, which brought with it adrenal issues and blood sugar handling issues, namely hypoglycemia and insulin resistance. Since all of this runs in the family, I researched all that I could and looked as far back into my family tree as possible. There was diabetes on my mother's side and undiagnosed autoimmune disease on my father's side. Plus, my cousins had Hashimoto's disease and were not diagnosed until the fifth decade of life, just like me.

They're So Entwined

The symptoms of thyroid conditions can sometimes be confused with diabetes symptoms. They can also be mistakenly attributed to other circumstances. In his blog, diabetes journalist David Mendosa wrote the following about his hypothyroidism diagnosis:

> My feet were cold most of the time. Even when I wore thick woollen socks to bed my feet were often so uncomfortable that they interfered with my sleep.
>
> Since I have diabetes, I assumed that my problem was that I had one of the most common complications of our condition, peripheral neuropathy. So I focused all the more on controlling my blood glucose levels in hopes of reversing my problem someday.
>
> Good strategy in general. But worse than useless when the assumption is faulty.
>
> My problem is hypothyroidism...
>
> But different people have different symptoms, and some people don't have any of them. "Hypothyroidism is more common than you would believe, and millions of people are currently hypothyroid and diabetic and don't know it," says James Norman, MD...
>
> Hypothyroidism is an endocrine condition—just like diabetes is. That fact led me to wonder if people with diabetes are more likely to have hypothyroidism than most people. Studies, in fact, show that it is.[6]

My maternal grandmother was a severe diabetic, and she lost her sight and a limb to this dreaded disease. Looking at her pictures as I write this book, I can see that she had all of the facial characteristics of a hypothyroid patient. She had a round, puffy face, was overweight, had low moods, and always seemed unhappy. She endured more stress than most people could ever imagine during the years of the Great Depression, with five children and a husband who came home from the war only to make another child. She was destitute, and she was ashamed of her lot in life. She struggled with her health for most of her life. She had the face of thyroid disease with diabetes as a traveling companion.

Could it be that treating her thyroid back then could have spared my grandmother much of her suffering? Could a thyroid diagnosis and treatment have prevented her diabetes from progressing to the point of blindness? This I will never know. But I do know that your endocrine system is interconnected. If one endocrine gland is under attack or is low functioning, the other endocrine glands will pay a price. This is especially true if your thyroid issue is autoimmune.

In my journey I devoured all of the research and studies I could possibly digest. Along the way, one fact that I came across over and over again was that people who have type 1 diabetes are more likely than others to develop an autoimmune thyroid condition.

What's more, the occurrence of thyroid disease of all types (hypo, hyper, or autoimmune) may be as high as 30 percent in people diagnosed with type 1 diabetes. Women are more at risk than men, whether they are diabetic or not; women are five to eight times more likely than men to develop thyroid disease.[7]

Diabetes and thyroid disease are often traveling companions, with autoimmunity driving the bus. Autoimmune diseases often run in families. Unfortunately my daughters and I have experienced autoimmunity with our diagnosis of Hashimoto's and all of its unpleasant symptoms. Thinking back on my maternal grandmother, who may have had undiagnosed thyroid problems—she certainly *was* a diabetic!

What we know now is that thyroid disease may occur many years before a type 1 diabetes diagnosis. In the past many if not most diabetic patients were found to have thyroid issues *after* receiving their diagnosis of diabetes.

If you remember how important blood sugar balance is to your endocrine system, you can certainly see that the entire endocrine system must be working like a team of horses. If one horse or endocrine gland gets weakened, the entire team must pick up the slack. Eventually each and every horse or endocrine gland gets overworked. This sets the stage for autoimmunity, which includes diabetes, thyroid disease, and adrenal involvement.

The purpose of this book is to help you get diagnosed sooner rather than later. Untreated thyroid disease can dramatically affect your blood sugar levels and just may be an underlying factor in your developing type 1 diabetes. If you are having a lot of trouble controlling your blood sugar right now, please have your thyroid checked!

If you have already been diagnosed with type 1 diabetes and are having an especially difficult time keeping your sugar under control and at acceptable levels—for example, if your blood sugar runs too low—it may be a sign of hypothyroidism. Conversely, if your blood sugar runs in the high range, you may have undiagnosed hyperthyroidism.

My point here is, be *aware*. If you have diabetes, you are at risk for thyroid disease, and if you have thyroid disease, you are at risk for diabetes. Do not let your health-care provider chalk up tiredness and a feeling of unwellness to "just your diabetes" and tell you that "you will have to live with it."

As I mentioned earlier, thyroid disease is insidious. Symptoms can come and go for decades, leaving your thyroid so damaged from the autoimmune assault that your symptoms can no longer be ignored. By that time you may also find yourself hearing these three words: "You have diabetes."

To be forewarned is to be forearmed. As you can see, getting thyroid disease diagnosed and properly managed is imperative when it comes to blood sugar matters.

IT'S REALLY COMPLICATED

When it comes to blood sugar and thyroid disease, there are layers upon layers that need to be addressed. This includes balancing all other endocrine glands because they work in symphony. Clinical studies show that hypothyroidism increases insulin secretion. By treating your thyroid condition, you may normalize your insulin production and thereby prevent diabetes.[8] Hashimoto's is so much more than a thyroid problem; it is a multisystem problem that can only be solved with a multisystem approach.

Chapter 8

THE THYROID AND AUTOIMMUNITY

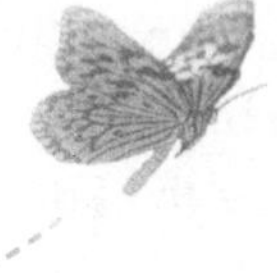

SOMETHING YOU NEED to understand about thyroid conditions is that most cases are autoimmune. I learned the hard way that even though my thyroid gland was removed surgically, and even though my daughter had her thyroid removed as well, autoimmunity did not abate for either of us. We also did not realize that because autoimmunity had taken hold first by launching an attack on the thyroid, we were at greater risk of developing additional autoimmune disorders such as lupus and rheumatoid arthritis. As a matter of fact, I did develop rheumatoid arthritis antibodies and began to have "flares" during this bewildering time.

Luckily I soon learned I would have to apply all that I had studied over the past twenty-five years in a huge way. I had to save my daughters and myself from the specter of autoimmunity, which is considered a life sentence of pain.

The underlying causes, or "triggers," had to be found; most of the time these are a combo of adrenal dysfunction, "leaky gut," food allergies, stress, stealthy infections, and toxicity due to your body's poor ability to detoxify. In the context of addressing your thyroid disease, medication is one way to skin this cat. Since most cases deal with an autoimmune etiology, you must focus on your immune system.

Today autoimmune thyroid disease is on the rise, and sadly it is underdiagnosed. When we talk about autoimmune thyroid disease, we think of Hashimoto's thyroiditis and Graves' disease. Hashimoto's is the most common autoimmune thyroid disease. It is harder to diagnose, and you know by now it is the disease that so affected my life and the lives of my two daughters that we almost gave up. This is why I have chosen to focus on Hashimoto's—or "Hashi's"—in this book, as it is the most elusive and undetected. Once it is finally detected, it is largely mismanaged by both conventional and alternative professionals.

But Graves' disease is the other form of autoimmune thyroiditis. Whereas Hashi's is a hypothyroid, or underfunctioning, autoimmune disorder, Graves' disease is the opposite—a hyperthyroid, or overfunctioning, autoimmune disorder. The calling card of Graves' disease is hard to miss with its literal "eye-popping" symptoms, heart palpitations, trembling, fast pulse, nervousness, night sweats, and weight loss.

No matter which of these two diseases you have, it is disheartening to find out your body is attacking itself, creating an autoimmune disease that seeks to destroy your thyroid gland, and along with it, your quality of life. It is also quite alarming to find out that your body believes a gland or organ in your own body is a foreign invader, which is really what happens with an autoimmune disease.

What makes it even more frightening is that once you have one autoimmune condition, you're likely to have more. A person with long-standing, untreated Hashi's can face a progression of assaults against other organ systems. One example is developing pernicious anemia, where the immune system attacks the stomach's intrinsic factor so that B_{12} cannot be properly absorbed. This is a prime case where a doctor would typically a give B_{12} shot, never going deeper into the cause. The pancreas may also be attacked when the immune system launches an assault on the islet cells within the gland, causing type 1 diabetes.

As time goes on and the true trigger is not addressed, autoimmunity can spread its inflammation like a little brush fire, sending sparks to your joints, skin, lungs, kidneys, and even your brain. Soon, though, your entire body can become engulfed in the flames of full-blown autoimmunity.

Know What You Have

It is critically important to find out early if your thyroid symptoms are in actuality an autoimmune disease. How do you find out whether your symptoms relate to a straightforward case of hypothyroidism or actually indicate an autoimmune disease like Hashimoto's?

The answer is *antibodies*.

With a straightforward case of hypothyroidism, you will have an elevated TSH with no antibodies. If you fall into this category, you will be prescribed a thyroid hormone replacement. There are also some cases where natural supplements can help to improve your TSH levels, making medication unnecessary. But if you *do* have antibodies, this indicates an autoimmune disease at work, which requires alternative treatment.

Another twist in the elusive diagnostic processes that even the best of physicians may not realize is that some Hashimoto's sufferers' immune systems may be so depressed that they cannot even produce antibodies. Additionally, if you have symptoms of hyperthyroidism and hypothyroidism, you should suspect Hashimoto's despite normal antibody levels. If you are taking an iodine supplement and your symptoms intensify, this is a very good clue that you are dealing with Hashimoto's, and you should stop taking it entirely or decrease your dose and proceed with caution. (More about iodine later in this chapter.)

DIAGNOSING AUTOIMMUNITY

If you are diagnosed with autoimmune disease of any kind, it can be frustrating! It is important for you to become your own advocate and speak up if you are not satisfied with the medical advice that you have been given. Steps must be taken to get to the root of your autoimmunity, and you will need a doctor who will partner with you to help you do just that. Remember to PUSH!

Let's look at the factors that go into an autoimmunity diagnosis and treatment.

Triggers

A trigger can be anything that moves the autoimmune needle forward. Possible triggers include gluten, dairy, stress (divorce, death in the family, abuse, job loss, trouble with a child, being a caregiver, etc.), blood sugar issues, genetically modified foods, pesticides, herbicides, insecticides, heavy metals, chronic toxin exposure, viruses, infections, BPA in plastic, alcohol, prescription medications, and mold exposure.

Genes

Certain genes predispose our immune systems to misfire. But please know that having a gene does *not* equal a diagnosis. For example, I could have the gene for breast cancer, but with the right lifestyle choices I could save myself a diagnosis. On the contrary, I might not have the gene for breast cancer, but if I choose to drink in excess, smoke, and not manage stress well, I could end up with breast cancer. Just because you inherit a gene doesn't make you a prime candidate for a disease. I am telling you that autoimmune disease is a real wake-up call, whether you have a genetic predisposition or not. Again, genes do not have to express. The amount of autoimmunity in your family tree is very important to know, as it can alert you to do the things I have outlined here to help you possibly circumvent autoimmunity in yourself and your loved ones. If you are diagnosed with autoimmune thyroid disease, taking these steps will help you to manage the symptoms and focus on all of the areas that broke down or were breached. These suggestions will help support you the rest of your life.

Toxins

Toxins can play a part in autoimmunity. Limit use of plastics in cooking and especially when you drink hot beverages. Use glass in cooking and to drink from as much as possible. Look at the ingredients in your skin care and hair care products. If you wear makeup, switch to products that are free of chemicals and preservatives such as parabens. If you smoke, it is time to stop. Heavy metals are implicated in the constellation of causative factors of autoimmune disease. You may have a simple blood test to screen for levels of heavy metals such as lead and mercury. Mercury fillings and root canals that have not healed properly or still harbor infection can "stir up" autoimmunity. Consider having mercury amalgam fillings removed (make sure this is done according to proper protocol). Seek out an endodontist to check any root canals you may have for possible failure. Chronic infections can be "stealthy," in that they can become entrenched and elude detection for years, leaving you vulnerable to inflammation from your immune system's constant attempt to fight an oftentimes "cell wall deficient" bacteria.

Inflammation

Since inflammation is the cause of all diseases, not just the autoimmune variety, and since autoimmune disease has increased thirtyfold over the past thirty years, you have to wonder where the root cause lies. More and more often the answer is "leaky gut," where food, proteins, and bacteria "leak" into the bloodstream, causing inflammation all over.

Eighty percent of your immunity resides in your gut. Healthy intestinal flora (probiotics) keep your intestinal lining healthy. Taking a good source of probiotics will help restock your intestinal pond with the "good guys," healthy bacteria.

Work on repairing "leaky gut" first by removing gluten, sugars, legumes, caffeine, soy, and refined and fried foods. Limit or eliminate steroids, NSAIDS, and antibiotics. A healthy gut lining is a good barrier between your bloodstream and your intestinal tract. If your gut is inflamed from gluten or other allergenic food, undigested food will "leak" into your bloodstream and cause constant stimulation and inflammation of your immune system as it tries to defend itself from the perceived invader (your food). This leads to system malfunction and ultimately causes autoimmune disease.

Diet

Another important thing to address is diet. It is important to eat lean protein–based foods and avoid going more than three hours between meals. This will help to balance your blood sugar, which in turn will help you to avoid insulin and hormone fluctuations. These peaks and valleys are very hard on your immune system.

You need to be on an elimination diet. If you test positive for thyroid antibodies, you need to stay off gluten, dairy, and soy for life. Other foods you should initially avoid are eggs, corn, nightshades (i.e., tomatoes, peppers, eggplant, potatoes), and most grains except for rice. Take probiotics if you have a history of antibiotic use.

Liver health is important in regard to metabolizing antibodies. Drinking one glass of water with fresh lemon juice can help keep your liver cleansed during the restoration process.

Vitamins and supplements

If you find that you have TPO and/or TgAb (antibodies), it is important that you begin supplementation with vitamin D, as studies have found that over 90 percent of people with autoimmune thyroid disease have a genetic defect that affects their ability to process vitamin D.[1] This means that if you have Hashi's or any other autoimmune disease, you will need higher amounts of vitamin D to recover and maintain your health.

Have your vitamin D levels tested often to make sure that you are being optimized. The usual dosage is 5,000 IUs or more daily.

Because of leaky gut issues that go hand and hand with autoimmunity, a B_{12} deficiency may be causing anemia. Both of my daughters experienced this. Sublingual B_{12} (1 mg) taken daily will help rectify the situation.

Desiccated thyroid hormone medication, such as Armour, Nature-Throid, or Westhroid, contains T4, T3, T2, and T1, just like the thyroid gland in the body produces (as opposed to Synthroid, which only contains T4).

Stress

I would be remiss if I left out the last and probably most important part of calming your immune system back down, causing the attack to abate. If you find that you do in fact have autoimmune thyroid disease, you now know that it is more of an immune system disease than a thyroid condition. Your thyroid is the victim of your immunity run wild. Now more than any other time in your life, you must work on dealing with your levels of stress. Stress causes your adrenal health to suffer, and as you have learned, the thyroid-adrenal connection is strong. Long-term stress and exhausted adrenals can also affect your gut's integrity.

It is time to let go of what no longer serves your life in a healthy way. If you feel that a relationship or a job is draining the very life out of you, it is. If you have buried hurt deep inside, now is the time to unearth it, or it may bury you in autoimmune issues. Thyroid disease slows your life down. This is especially true when it is autoimmune thyroid disease. The pains, the fatigue, the anxiety, and every other symptom that rides along can make life hard to bear. I know. I have been there. I have also witnessed this in both of my daughters.

Treating autoimmunity

To summarize, if you have autoimmune thyroid disease—or any autoimmune disease, for that matter—do the following:

1. Check for hidden food allergies with an IgG (Immunoglobulin G) blood test. Many people with autoimmunity have food allergies. The IgG blood test will help find the offending foods that are contributing to the autoimmune assault.
2. Have your doctor test you for stealth infections such as Lyme disease, viruses such as EBV (Epstein-Barr virus), mycoplasma, and yeast overgrowth.

3. Make exercise a part of your day, even if it is only taking a short walk. Exercise is a natural anti-inflammatory!
4. Heavy metals often play a part in autoimmunity, so get tested for heavy metal toxicity.
5. Work on fixing your gut health. Autoimmunity begins in the gut. Probiotics are a must!
6. Ask your doctor to check you for celiac disease by running a gliadin antibody blood test.
7. If your doctor is *not* a functional medicine doctor, seek one out, or find one that will partner with your current physician to maximize your care.
8. Stress makes all autoimmune diseases worse. Practice deep breathing several times daily, schedule regular massages, take a yoga class, and take long walks alone to commune with God.
9. Take fish oil, vitamin D, vitamin C, and a good quality probiotic each and every day. These are immune system–calming nutrients that will help your body come back into balance.

I am giving you vital information that will save you from years of wandering from doctor to doctor, spending thousands of dollars and hundreds of hours to no avail. If you follow the above steps, the assault on your thyroid and the rest of your body will decrease and ultimately cease! Your answer is on this page. If you find and address the underlying causes of your illness, you will begin to experience vibrant health once more.

DIAGNOSING HASHIMOTO'S THYROIDITIS

Hypothyroidism and Hashimoto's thyroid disease look and act the same. They have identical symptoms, such as the following:

- Neck swelling
- Coarse voice
- Mind issues, such as brain fog and poor memory and concentration
- Dry, cracking skin
- Brittle nails
- Excessive hair loss
- Constipation
- Muscle and joint pain
- Carpal tunnel syndrome or tendonitis
- Weight gain
- Inability to lose weight
- Mood swings
- Anxiety and/or depression
- PMS
- Irregular periods
- Low sex drive
- Fatigue best described as "bone tired"

With all these factors at play, you see why this often-masked villain sends people from one specialist to another in hope of addressing each and every one. Since Hashimoto's and hypothyroidism have the same symptoms, I cannot stress enough that you must find out if what you are really dealing with is Hashimoto's rather than straightforward hypothyroidism. If you have Hashi's, you are in a battle to take back your body from an immune system run amok.

It's tricky.

Hashimoto's can go undetected for decades; it happened to me. Unfortunately I am not alone. A friend of mine frantically went to a cardiologist, a dietician, a psychologist, and her long-time family primary care physician. She had no idea her thyroid was under attack. She was assured by her doctor and her normal TSH reading that her thyroid was functioning just fine. Without having her antibodies tested sooner, she went for decades undiagnosed, and as a result she experienced many uncomfortable symptoms that robbed her of her ability to experience life to its fullest. Her world became very small as she "begged off" from many social events due to her yet-to-be-diagnosed illness. I know all too well the frustration and anguish associated with this disease and the arduous task of getting to a diagnosis.

She went to four different doctors. Her weight and cholesterol increased, her mood swings became uncontrollable, and she became severely anxious and depressed. One doctor convinced her that she needed anxiety medication. The doctors only relied on her TSH levels; if the levels were in the normal range, they didn't think her concerns were thyroid related. She then had her antibody tests run, per my suggestion. Bingo! She too had Hashimoto's! The doctors missed it!

I urged my friend's sister to have her thyroid antibodies

checked because she was also very frustrated. It took almost thirty years for the doctors to diagnose her with Hashimoto's. It started with a positive serum RA (blood test for rheumatoid arthritis). She suffered with muscle aches, severe hip pain, and headaches. Almost all the doctors were dismissive and made her feel downright crazy. After undergoing an MRI after a car accident, doctors found that all that remained of her thyroid was a ragged left lobe. The right lobe had been destroyed after all the years of being undiagnosed and untreated for Hashimoto's. Since her diagnosis, and with the proper thyroid medication, she has slept well with no aches and pains except for mild hip pain, and she is very happy to report that her constipation is a thing of the past!

Two antibody tests can save you more than just years spent going from doctor to doctor and the physical and financial tolls that it takes; these two tests can possibly save your life.

It is important to note that you can have a perfectly normal TSH level and still have Hashimoto's. That was true in my case. That is why I was undiagnosed for decades. A simple antibody test could have saved me from years of suffering from one autoimmune symptom after another. Knowing that I had Hashimoto's sooner would have saved my daughters from having to deal with the fatigue, insomnia, anxiety, headaches, dizziness, and so much more. My daughters were as sidelined as I was, all because the proper tests were not performed.

You also need to know that many doctors do not believe in testing you for antibodies if your TSH is within normal limits. They feel that even if you do have antibodies, the treatment is the same. They either give you thyroid hormones to help support your thyroid while your body continues its attack against it, or they tell you to wait until your thyroid is destroyed before they give you any thyroid medication. Blessed you are if you can get to a health-care provider that knows the difference between hypothyroidism and autoimmune thyroid disease! That doctor is worth his or her weight in gold.

It's Hashimoto's—now what?

When I received the diagnosis of Hashimoto's thyroiditis, it was a scary time, compounded by the fact that my two daughters had it as well. It is was hard to come to the realization that our bodies' immune systems, which were designed to protect us, were attacking our thyroid cells. Little did we know then that its attack—with all of its life-disrupting and life-altering symptoms—would for us eventually become papillary thyroid cancer.

Believe me, trying to manage your day-to-day life without a thyroid and dealing with the autoimmune attacks that go on afterward is no walk in the park. My main focus and goal was to help calm the autoimmune attack while we struggled to find just the right thyroid hormone medication dose and the correct dietary changes, which included focusing on healing our leaky gut issues.

Stress management was crucial and will always be. This encompassed letting go of past hurts and forgiving ourselves and others. All of these components, plus the right supplements, helped our systems recover from years of metabolic issues and autoimmune assault.

When I was diagnosed with Hashimoto's, I soon came to realize that I was in a fight to save not only my thyroid but my entire body. This was a frightening thought and one that played on my mind each and every day. But I didn't know that this attack against my thyroid gland would eventually lead to life-disrupting metabolic symptoms and an increased risk of thyroid cancer.

Even more frightening was the treatment plan—or lack thereof—from traditional medicine. "Take this synthetic thyroid medicine, and poof! You'll be all better. Not better? Well, let's just take that nasty thyroid out! There you go. All better! Still not better? I'm sorry, I can't help you." The patient's life is spent trying to find optimal thyroid hormone replacement.

I have come to believe that traditional medicine does not have the answers. Many of you who are reading this have come to the same belief, and I feel your pain—*literally*. But there is good news here. You *can* get well. I believe you *can* normalize your thyroid function, and you *can* get rid of or lower your thyroid antibodies significantly! All you have to do is think outside of the box—or should I say, the doctor's waiting room, where patients virtually spend years waiting.

It is important here to remember that Hashimoto's is more than a thyroid condition. It is an autoimmune disease. Again, having one autoimmune disease sets the stage for more. This means you must do all that you can to get your thyroid antibody levels down, which will lessen the attack on your thyroid, calm your immune system, and possibly spare you from more autoimmune disease.

Uncover the reason

Now we are going to dive deep into the murky waters of autoimmunity. I hope to help you see more clearly how important it is to be proactive in terms of taking the "tack" out of your immune system's attack on your body. The "tack" I refer to here is the trigger, much like a thorn in a lion's paw or a splinter in your finger. It's about answering the question, what is it that has caused your immune system to launch an attack against your thyroid?

Once you have an autoimmune issue like Hashi's, your

job is to find out why. Hashimoto's thyroiditis risk factors include the following:

- Insulin resistance
- Polycystic ovary syndrome (PCOS)
- Vitamin D deficiency
- Chronic infection
- Estrogen fluctuations
- Heavy metal exposure
- Environmental pollutants
- Gluten intolerance
- Chronic inflammation

Hashimoto's runs in families and is five to eight times more common in women.[2] Therefore, I would urge all of you with Hashimoto's and/or hypothyroidism to encourage your daughters, sisters, mothers, aunts, and grandmothers to get tested, especially if they are in the age range of puberty, pregnancy, or perimenopause, the three most common times for thyroid hormone abnormalities to surface. Also, just because the condition is more common in women, this does not mean that men are not affected. I would urge you to have your male family members tested as well. Getting your diagnosis is the first step!

Given the fact that about 90 percent of all cases of hypothyroid disease are autoimmune,[3] I want to give you a heads-up on what to look for so you can be spared decades of suffering.

There are certain physiological conditions that can set the stage for Hashimoto's disease. These are gluten intolerance, estrogen surges, insulin resistance, polycystic ovary syndrome (PCOS), vitamin D deficiency, environmental toxicity, chronic infections, inflammation, and of course, genetic susceptibility. But what causes your genes to "turn on" the autoimmune response can be different from what turned on mine. Even so, here are some common indicators.

Stress

I would have to say that a huge predictor is stress. There is no doubt that stress plays a huge part in the development or triggering of autoimmune disease. Stress taxes your adrenal glands, so it is no wonder that it starts the autoimmune parade.

This was true in my case and in the cases of all of the women I have interviewed since and helped move to the diagnosis sooner rather than later. Many of these women had gone through a trauma of some kind—the death of a family member, a painful divorce, problems with children, or great financial difficulty. I put it this way: Your body follows how your mind and emotions react to stress. What eats at you mentally will in turn eat away at your body in the form of autoimmune disease.

Gluten intolerance

Many studies from several countries show a very strong link between Hashimoto's disease and gluten intolerance. Gluten intolerance is a huge causative agent that contributes to the weakening of your immune barrier, namely your digestive tract.

Your digestive tract is the very seat of your immune system. If you add sugar-laden, processed, and refined foods, antibiotics, steroids, and NSAID use, the immune barrier in your gut is breached and it becomes porous, or leaky, hence the term "leaky gut." I have mentioned leaky gut already, so you are correct in assuming it is extremely important to make that priority one in your battle to make your autoimmunity retreat.

You should also know that if your gut's integrity has been impaired and has become "leaky," it will allow undigested food particles, bacteria, and harmful substances to leak back into your bloodstream. Once these substances have leaked back in, your immune system treats them as invaders called antigens.

This is where the trouble really begins. Your immune system does only what God designed it to do—attack the invaders! What's more, once your gut's barrier is compromised, this will happen every time you eat. Gluten causes inflammation each and every time you eat it. It is interesting to know that with Hashimoto's, the attack on your thyroid happens as a result of your immune system confusing your thyroid gland with the gluten that leaked through your gut. This happens because gluten molecules very closely resemble thyroid tissue.

The big tip for you at this point is to remove wheat gluten from your diet. It is becoming common knowledge that the wheat we now eat is not the same wheat as our grandparents ate. In today's world wheat has been genetically modified, increasing its number of genes, which results in more gluten in our wheat than ever before. More and more people are being diagnosed with autoimmune thyroid disease since the advent of genetically modified organisms (GMOs), and Hashi's seems to have a strong connection to this "new wheat gluten."

Again, since a strong link has been found between gluten and its inflammatory effect on the gut, which is where most of our immunity resides, it is crucial to eliminate gluten if you have positive antibodies, and especially if you have Hashimoto's disease. We'll discuss this further in chapter 13.

Iodine—yes or no?

Once I found out that I had Hashimoto's thyroiditis, I quickly began to take Iodoral 50 mg (iodine). My symptoms got much worse, and the autoimmune attack on my thyroid increased! What I did not know then is that iodine and selenium, when taken together, can make a wonderful difference!

THE BACKSTORY

Years ago, researchers discovered that iodine deficiency was the most common cause of hypothyroidism worldwide. This prompted health authorities from all over the world to add iodine to table salt. Now, while this proved effective for correcting iodine deficiency, something unexpected and undesirable happened. Cases of autoimmune thyroid disease began to rise! It was later found that if you increase iodine intake, it can cause an autoimmune attack on the thyroid gland, because iodine reduces the action of an enzyme called thyroid peroxidase, or TPO, which is essential for optimal thyroid health.

Here's more. Restricting iodine can actually reverse hypothyroidism, according to one study where 78 percent of patients with Hashimoto's recovered perfectly normal thyroid function by iodine restriction alone.[4]

How do we make sense of this information? I have done the work for you—and believe me, it took years. It appears that iodine may cause a problem for people with Hashimoto's or other autoimmune issues who have a selenium deficiency.

Studies show that selenium can protect you against the effects of iodine toxicity, which in turn prevents the triggering and flaring of autoimmunity. What does all of this mean? Simply that you are armed with yet another bit of information that can positively affect your recovery. When your doctor wants to test you for Hashimoto's, be sure to ask him to test your iodine levels as well. If your iodine levels come back low or on the low side of normal, this is your green light to start a trial of iodine and selenium to see if your symptoms improve. Remember, managing autoimmune thyroid issues is not one size fits all. There are variables, and some people will not be able to take a small dose of iodine even if they take it with selenium.

Be sure to work with a health-care provider that understands iodine testing and replacement—preferably a functional medicine doctor, who will know the best way to test for iodine deficiency. Blood tests are not always accurate, so functional medicine doctors often use a twenty-four-hour urine loading test. This test involves giving you a large dose of iodine and then collecting your urine for the next twenty-four hours. At the end of the twenty-four-hour time period, the level of iodine in your urine is measured. If it is lower than expected, it means that you are indeed deficient and your body held on to the iodine it needed.

If you have trouble finding a health-care provider who will test you, you may simply do your own trial by taking a low-dose kelp tablet that contains 325 mcg of iodine with 200 mcg of selenium daily to offset any potentially uncomfortable issues. This is very important, especially if you have Hashimoto's. If you feel worse (hyper, headache, more aches and pains), then iodine is not for you. Conversely, if you feel better, you might have found another piece to your wellness puzzle.

Be aware that some well-meaning physicians believe in starting all thyroid patients on iodine, and at high doses. I had this experience, and it was *not* pleasant; my symptoms greatly intensified. Selenium was never mentioned. In addition, high doses of iodine can raise your TSH so it will appear that your hypothyroidism and/or autoimmunity is getting worse!

Please make sure to ask if your health-care provider understands the importance of the iodine and selenium relationship. It will help to spare you from taking a giant step backward. You *are* going forward. Backward is no longer an option.

DIAGNOSING GRAVES' DISEASE

Like Hashimoto's disease, Graves' disease is an autoimmune disease where antibodies attack the thyroid gland. But in the case of Graves', the attack causes an increase in thyroid hormone production, making the body use energy faster than it normally would.

Graves' disease, which was discovered in 1835 by Irish physician Robert J. Graves, is the main cause of hyperthyroidism. The symptoms of Graves' are quite troubling, to say the least. Weight loss, sweating, palpitations, and anxiety are just a few of the symptoms that send people to the ER or urgent care before they receive their diagnosis.

As with other autoimmune issues, stress is considered a trigger that brings Graves' on suddenly. And like other autoimmune diseases, Graves' is thought to be linked to a bacterial or viral infection with a strong connection to *Yersinia enterocolitica,* which may be responsible for triggering antibodies.[5] Genetics also play a part, but stress seems to encourage genes to express, thereby opening the door to autoimmune disease.

Graves' patients must be properly managed so as not to experience the dreaded "thyroid storm" caused by a drastic increase in thyroid hormones. Symptoms include severe hypotension (low blood pressure), confusion, disorientation, fever, profuse sweating, and coma.

What are the symptoms of a thyroid on overdrive?

- Weight loss
- Hot flashes, increased sweating, or overheating
- Anxiety
- Rapid or irregular heartbeat
- Shortness of breath
- Muscle weakness
- Insomnia
- Frequent bowel movements or diarrhea
- Irregular menstrual cycles
- Tremors, particularly in the hands and feet.
- Irritability and moodiness
- Erectile dysfunction or reduced sex drive
- Swelling of the neck and protrusion of the eyes
- The skin on the shins and/or tops of the feet becomes thick and red

How is it diagnosed?

Just as with Hashimoto's disease, Graves' disease can be found by performing a simple, antibody-specific blood test that allows your doctor to examine specific thyroid hormone levels in your blood. In Graves' disease, your immune system creates thyroid stimulating immunoglobulins (TSIs) that cause your thyroid to grow and make more thyroid hormone than your body needs, which can make you feel as though you have had ten cups of coffee! Graves' can also be diagnosed with a thyroid scan. If your doctor decides that you must have a thyroid scan, you will be asked to swallow a small amount of radioactive iodine in a liquid or capsule form. The amount of iodine your thyroid gland takes up will then be measured. Low uptake suggests Hashimoto's thyroiditis, while high uptake suggests Graves' disease.

GRAVES' DISEASE AT A GLANCE: CAN IT BE TREATED?

The treatment goal for Graves' disease is to control your overactive thyroid. Drugs called beta-blockers are often used to control the uncomfortable and frightening symptoms of rapid heart rate, sweating, and anxiety, until the hyperthyroidism is controlled. Hyperthyroidism, or autoimmune Graves' disease, is traditionally treated with one or more of the following:

- Antithyroid medication, such as Propranolol (Inderal), Atenolol (Tenormin), Metoprolol (Lopressor, Toprol-XL), or Nadolol (Corgard): these medications are used to calm the symptoms of Graves', including rapid heart rate, shortness of breath, sweating, and tremors
- Radioactive iodine: otherwise known as RAI (radioactive thyroid ablation), this treatment will essentially "kill" the thyroid, requiring you to take thyroid hormone

replacement for the rest of your life to prevent hypothyroidism

- Surgery: having your thyroid partially or completely removed will require you to take thyroid replacement hormone for the rest of your life in order to prevent hypothyroidism

Diagnosing Hope

In this chapter you have learned about a few of the far-reaching effects the health of your thyroid has on your entire body. The butterfly-shaped gland in your neck is a formidable player in the intricate dance of human physiology. There is hope when it comes to reversing this process, but you have to do the work. Getting well and out of that cocoon like a butterfly…it is up to you.

Chapter 9

THE THYROID AND THE BRAIN

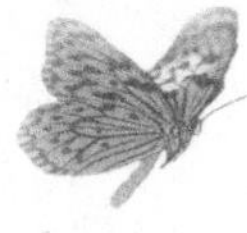

ONE OF THE most life-disrupting symptoms I experienced leading up to my diagnosis was anxiety. I experienced daily spells of "air hunger" (shortness of breath), feeling wired and tired, and severe panic attacks. I went to cardiologists, had stress tests performed, and sought out numerous physicians for help. None of them suspected thyroid disease.

Having an excess amount of thyroid hormone can make us extremely anxious, irritable, and on edge. This is one symptom commonly attributed to Graves' disease, but it can also crop up in Hashimoto's disease. In the early stages of Hashimoto's, the thyroid is under attack by the immune system. Thyroid cells are broken down, and they release thyroid hormones into the bloodstream. This causes thyroid hormone surges, or transient hyperthyroidism.

Anxiety, air hunger, panic attacks, sleepless nights, and heart palpitations controlled and ruined my life for almost twenty years. Little did I know back then that my thyroid was to blame. My experience is not uncommon, unfortunately, as each day I receive e-mails, texts, and instant messages from women who are desperate to find help for these symptoms.

You learned in the last chapter that most cases of hypothyroidism are autoimmune, which means that there is an all-out attack on that little butterfly-shaped gland in your neck twenty-four hours a day. When the attack is in progress, it causes your thyroid gland to release more thyroid hormone than your body is accustomed to into your bloodstream. The result? You feel wired, anxious, panicky, and short of breath. Thyroid hormones control everything, and when they are out of whack, they really show you who is the boss!

My goal is to get you to diagnosis quickly so you do not have to suffer for decades as my daughters and I did. With the proper thyroid medication (which we will discuss later) coupled with the tests and lifestyle and dietary changes you have learned so far, your angst will soon be a thing of the past. I am living proof!

Now I Know Why I Thanked God for GABA!

In my book *Breaking the Grip of Dangerous Emotions* I sang the praises of GABA (gamma-aminobutyric acid), a neurotransmitter I took in capsule form that calmed my panic attacks. It was a godsend—not only for me, but for thousands. It has been almost a decade since I wrote that book, and now I understand so much more about how GABA came to my rescue and helped me and thousands of others overcome feelings of anxiety and panic.

Technical but necessary information here: there is an enzyme called glutamic acid decarboxylase (GAD) that actually triggers the production of GABA (your brain's most calming neurotransmitter). Here is where it all came together for me, and it hopefully will for you. It is now known that some people develop an autoimmune reaction to GAD, meaning your immune system destroys it. The result? You cannot make enough GABA to keep your brain and body calm. Many people have given in to taking benzodiazepines like Xanax or Ativan or resorted to antidepressants to cope with GABA deficiency and GAD autoimmunity symptoms, which include OCD, vertigo, motion sickness, and facial tics, to name a few.

Another interesting discovery is that GAD autoimmunity and resultant GABA deficiency is common in people with celiac disease or gluten sensitivity. Gluten plays a big role in the battle to reverse or calm Hashimoto's disease. Gluten is strongly linked to all autoimmune illness, especially autoimmune thyroid disease.[1] This is another reason to be tested for gliadin antibodies to make sure you are not gluten intolerant. Your takeaway? If you can relate to what you have just read, eliminate gluten and all grains from your life, and watch your life change!

GLUTEN—ANOTHER CAUSE FOR WORRY

Adopting a gluten-free diet is an important first step in battling not only autoimmune thyroid disease but all autoimmune illnesses. It is still hard for me to accept that all of the years I spent cooking wonderful Italian pasta and baking breads, cakes, and pies for my family actually contributed to the autoimmunity of my two daughters and me. All three of us found out decades later that we had gliadin antibodies, meaning we were gluten intolerant or sensitive. This set the stage for our Hashimoto's to manifest. Today functional medicine doctors as well as myself strongly recommend eliminating all grains to help quell inflammation and keep flare-ups and anxiety at bay. I have personally found that it works and gives people the hope they are seeking in terms of recovery from this seemingly unrelenting specter called autoimmune thyroid disease.

In the context of this chapter on brain health and thyroid disease, I suggest you follow an anti-inflammatory autoimmune diet, which you will find in chapter 14.

Remember, people with Hashimoto's hypothyroidism are typically gluten intolerant, gluten triggers brain inflammation, and brain inflammation triggers anxiety due to deficient GABA.[2]

Got Brain Drain?

Since this book is dedicated to the health of your thyroid, we cannot forget about the brain. Your thyroid gland is a huge player in the health of your brain, as healthy thyroid function exerts a powerful protective effect on the brain. It's like they say, "A drain on the brain can make you feel insane."

Knowledge has increased concerning the factors that lead to poor thyroid health. Gut infections, adrenal fatigue, poor diet, and unstable blood sugar cause not only gut inflammation but also brain tissue inflammation, degeneration, and a deficiency of the precious neurotransmitters that help brain cells communicate with one another.

Your brain is chock full of thyroid hormone receptors. An underfunctioning thyroid gland can cause mental fogginess and/or forgetfulness. When low thyroid function slows down your metabolism, it slows down your brain function with it. If you are dealing with symptoms of anxiety or depression, you may have low levels of the two most important neurotransmitters: serotonin (inhibitory) and dopamine (excitatory). These two amino acids are critically important when it comes to a feeling of well-being. Research shows that deficiencies in either one of these master neurotransmitters can slow down or hamper the conversion of T4 to T3 and slow down your brain's communication with your thyroid.

If your dopamine is depleted, you will find yourself reaching for substances like caffeine, chocolate, and nicotine. This is because dopamine is the "feel good" neurotransmitter, and those substances do the job when you are deficient in dopamine. There is a downside, however, because while those substances elevate dopamine temporarily, long-term dependency on them creates a more severe dopamine deficit. This is important to note because out of all of the brain's neurotransmitters, dopamine has a very intimate relationship with your thyroid gland and its ability to keep you up and running at full speed, fully engaged in life.

MY MOTHER'S STORY

My mother had classic signs of autoimmune disease, such as rashes, fatigue, psoriasis, and gastrointestinal issues. She reached for sugar and caffeine with what can only be described as a crazed frenzy. She had to have sugar and caffeine. It made her "feel better." Looking back now at my mother's life, I know that she was dealing with autoimmunity. Of course it was hard for me to recognize when I was a child. It was hardly even recognized by physicians back then.

What I know now about my mother's unfortunate life is that she experienced extreme, unspeakable abuse as a child—matters that were never spoken of in her generation. She never shared any of her past with me when I asked her to tell me stories. All she said was that it was awful and she was ashamed and chose not to speak of it.

Everything crystallized for me when I came home from school one day and found her burning a photo of a man I did not recognize. As soon as I gazed at that image, he was gone, instantly up in smoke. I asked my mother who he was, and her abrupt answer was, "That's your grandfather." I was shocked. Why would she burn her father's picture, and why could I not see my own grandfather? I was only ten years old then.

Now that I am older and wiser, I understand what she had to endure at a very young age. But shortly after that day I saw my grandfather "go up in smoke," so to speak, my father unexpectedly drove away, never to return to my mother, my brother, or me again.

My mother changed as the next few years passed. She worked hard to support us, but she became progressively moody. She became irrational at times and forgetful, and she struck out at me when I tried to help. It was hurtful, but I figured it was the stress that she was under trying to support us with no support from my father.

During that time she refused to see a doctor. She said she was fine and became agitated and paranoid when I asked her to come with me to the doctor for a checkup. She still craved sugar, caffeine, chocolate, and pastries over healthy food.

As another decade passed she became more and more argumentative and forgetful. She started losing things more frequently. She asked me questions about my children's names. She left food out for a week at a time and argued it was fine to do so. She stopped bathing, grooming, and calling me.

She was very hard to deal with, but I also knew love deals with all, so I did the best I could to care for her.

I somehow got her to see a neurologist—and believe me, it was no easy feat. Wouldn't you know it, the doctor's first question was, "Honey, do you have thyroid disease?" At that time, I thought it was a very strange question for her to ask. But in retrospect, this neurologist was correct to ask that very important question. She gave my mother a series of tests to check her mental ability, memory, recall, and so forth. My mother passed all of the tests. Next, the doctor ran blood work to check for thyroid issues, which she hoped to follow with a brain scan. However, my mother refused, no matter how much we both tried to reason with her that day. The doctor told me to bring her back another day so we could get the blood work results and do the brain scan. She told me that we had to see if this was a thyroid disease or Alzheimer's dementia.

My mother never wanted the blood results, and I did not have permission at that time to access the test results. She was very secretive and private, and she was becoming more suspicious of everyone, including me.

One more decade passed, and my mother kept declining in her ability to reason soundly. Finally I had to step in and do an intervention for her own good. Tests were finally run—and the results? Hashimoto's thyroiditis and advanced dementia. Sadly my mother passed away in 2012 from this insidious condition.

My dear mother had Hashimoto's disease and did not find out until she was seventy-two, when she was diagnosed with Alzheimer's disease. It was horrible to watch her slip away into the long good-bye of Alzheimer's. In earlier years conventional medicine really did not dig deep. The signs were there, but finding autoimmunity in the '70s was often described as a genius of diagnostic ability. Physicians did not focus on the gut-autoimmune-brain connection then. My mother went to her grave with autoimmune thyroid disease that ultimately destroyed her ability to reason or recognize her family. May she finally rest in peace.

Brain Aging, Brain Fog, and the Thyroid

According to Dr. Datis Kharrazian DHSc, DC, MS:

> If you're managing your Hashimoto's yet still waiting for your depression to lift and your memory to return, you could be suffering from the beginning of a brain

> breakdown. Scientists call it accelerated brain aging, and it's critical you know about it.[3]

He goes on to say:

> Researchers have found Hashimoto's and hypothyroidism increase the risk of developing Parkinson's or Alzheimer's disease. In fact, accelerated brain degeneration is one of the most severe consequences of poorly managed Hashimoto's hypothyroidism.[4]

What I know now is that an unsupported thyroid condition guarantees a measure of brain degeneration in time. I am grateful that I have found this extremely important thyroid-brain connection so that I can be proactive in terms of my brain health, my daughters' brain health, and your brain health. We are now forewarned, so we are forearmed.

Since poor thyroid health impacts all of your brain cells or neurotransmitters, it can lead to a myriad of symptoms. For example:

- Foggy head caused by a lack of sleep
- Low blood sugar
- Seasonal allergies
- Food allergies
- Dehydration
- Electrolyte imbalance after heavy exercise

When a woman reaches the menopausal years of life, she often faces a lot of losses. She loses her children to empty nest syndrome, one or both parents to death, her marriage may fail, her sight may grow dim, and her memory may start to fail as her hormone levels plummet.

While all of these things can cause a woman to feel unwell, one symptom that women hate is "brain fog," which can be a symptom of menopause *or* thyroid disease. Other causes include Lyme disease, depression, sex hormone depletion, fibromyalgia, or substance abuse. Medications and treatments such as chemotherapy can also cause cloudy brains.

Whatever the cause, a woman who experiences brain fog feels dull, like she is trying to think through oatmeal. And it is tiring.

It is interesting to note that many women experience thyroid issues at menopause. Think of how many women in the past, including our own mothers, could have lived better-quality lives if only they had their thyroids checked, tested, and treated optimally. If you are in your menopausal years and are experiencing brain fog, please have your thyroid checked, especially if thyroid issues or autoimmunity runs in your family! You will read more about menopause and your thyroid in the next chapter.

Losing your mental sharpness is considered a normal part of aging, but I do not believe you should simply accept it as a consequence of growing older. What symptoms alert you to the possibility that your thyroid health is affecting your brain and may be setting the stage for neurodegenerative disease?

First, there is dopamine deficiency, the symptoms of which include:

- Anger and aggression when under stress
- Feelings of hopelessness
- Self-destructive thoughts
- Inability to handle stress
- Distractibility

- Low libido
- Losing your temper inappropriately
- Inability to finish assigned tasks
- Desire to "cocoon" from others
- Unnatural lack of concern for family and friends

And then there is serotonin deficiency, which can include:

- Loss of pleasure
- Inner tension
- Feelings of rage
- Depression
- Not enjoying favorite foods
- Sensitivity to pain
- Difficulty falling asleep and staying asleep
- Inappropriate anger
- Loss of zest for life

If you can relate to any of these symptoms, it is important to stop the inflammation. Fix your gut. Address the stress that is weakening your adrenal glands. Change your diet by eliminating gluten, sugar, and refined foods, and limit antibiotic use. As we learned in the last chapter, all of these things trigger autoimmunity.

As I look back over the previous decades of my life, I remember symptoms that I can now attribute to the mental changes that are hallmarks of low thyroid function. I felt as though I had to think through oatmeal. My head felt like it was full of cotton, and it became harder to concentrate when I tried to read research articles. I also noticed that my handwriting began to change, and I also had to *really* think before I tried to write my name, or anyone else's, for that matter. After my Hashimoto's diagnosis, I read all I could and found that these are *very* common symptoms. They are subtle at first, as with my experience, but as time marches on, the symptoms march right along with more and more intensity. You may find that adding, subtracting, and even figuring out correct change becomes difficult, and you have to continually double check everything you do.

More than 80 percent of people with low-grade hypothyroidism have impaired memory function, according to brain expert Daniel Amen, MD.[5]

It is estimated that one-third of all depression cases are directly related to thyroid imbalance, and 80 to 90 percent of postpartum depression is associated with thyroid abnormalities.[6] This was quite an eye opener for me, since I suffered from postpartum depression for eighteen months after the birth of my first child. It was a scary and bewildering experience for a young woman of twenty years old back in the late 1970s when physicians did not make the thyroid connection.

What a travesty it is that the neurological symptoms from which about 5 percent of all hypothyroidism patients suffer[7] are underestimated and many times completely ignored by scores of medical professionals. I know firsthand...I was one of them.

The brain symptoms that ride along as part of the thyroid disease picture are often chalked up to stress, anxiety, or depression. This disservice—which happens especially to women, who make up the majority of cases—is no longer acceptable! These distressing symptoms are life disrupting, and many women are given what I like to call "shut em' up pills" like antianxiety or antidepressant medication!

It takes finding a physician who is well versed or at least open to the idea that your thyroid is making your life hard to deal with and that your symptoms are real. Symptoms should not be "smothered away" with conventional medication, but rather *investigated* to see if the thyroid is the culprit from which these brain manifestations often spring!

You probably understand by now how especially important proper thyroid function is to the functioning of not only your brain but also to each and every cell of your body. It should be clear that many of the most debilitating and life-disrupting symptoms of hypothyroidism are directly related to brain function. If you are experiencing, anxiety, panic attacks, poor memory, brain fatigue, depression, forgetfulness, irritability, poor focus, clumsiness, and slowed thinking, it is time to check your thyroid. PUSH and push hard. Demand the right tests that you have learned about in this book (especially the thyroid antibody test). Remember that many of the brain symptoms you may be experiencing can be due to a poorly functioning thyroid!

When It's Good to Have a "Fat Head"

Depleted levels of the neurotransmitters serotonin, dopamine, and GABA are often present in hypothyroidism and lead to the depression, irritability, poor stress tolerance, and general anxiety that often prevail. The good news here is that there are nutrients that support and protect your brain from the effects of hypothyroidism. The omega-3 fatty acids DHA and EPA can be powerful when it comes to protecting your brain. They have been known to stop thyroid disease's effect on your brain by quelling inflammation and tissue deterioration, and by helping to prevent structural changes in the hippocampus, which is your brain's command center for mood and memory. Supplementing with omega-3 oils can be so powerful that it stops the effect of hypothyroidism on the brain. What's more, omega-3 fish oils increase the brain's total antioxidant capacity, which helps to insure brain function integrity.

When the thyroid is not functioning properly, especially due to inflammation from an autoimmune thyroid disease like Hashimoto's, the hippocampus becomes stressed and its functions deteriorate, which leads to depression, disorientation, and poor memory. This is linked with neurodegenerative illness such as Alzheimer's disease. Please note, however, that these same symptoms can also be found in hypothyroidism with inadequate omega-3 oils. If you find yourself forgetting where you parked your car at the mall, feeling disoriented when the grocery store rearranges its shelves, or taking longer to do things that used to take a couple of minutes (like ordering from a menu), and you have thyroid disease, I believe that taking a daily omega-3 DHA and EPA supplement will provide neurological protection against hypothyroidism-induced cognitive impairment.

I cannot stress this enough: anyone with hypothyroidism, especially autoimmune thyroid disease, must consider it imperative to take omega-3 daily in supplemental form to protect and wage war against the dreaded neurodegeneration caused by thyroid disease.

As for my dear mother…Nothing can soothe the cry from her "long good-bye," but with this knowledge, *we*—you and I—now have a chance to fight the neurodegenerative changes caused by a lifetime of undiagnosed and untreated thyroid disease. Knowledge is *power*!

Chapter 10

THE THYROID AND MENOPAUSE

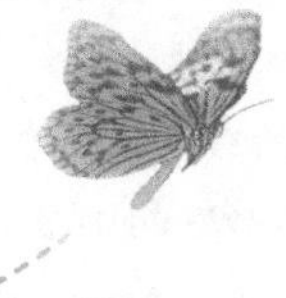

LITTLE DID I know that I would finally receive my diagnosis of Hashimoto's thyroiditis when I was in my menopausal years.

This was the diagnosis that had eluded me for decades. When I look back at my younger years, I remember there being strange findings in blood work that my doctors said were nothing, when in fact they were something. I had very low levels of progesterone, folate, vitamin D, and B vitamins. My body temp was 96.8, and my cholesterol was sky high. I had frequent strep infections, and many antibiotics were prescribed to me. I had systemic yeast infections as a result. But I was young and active, so no physician gave attention to the little things that turned out to be the big thing that robbed me of so much vitality and life.

As I grew older and became pregnant with my first child, I felt better than I ever had in my life. This was due to the increased levels of progesterone, which is the progestational hormone. It is also known as the hormone of well-being—and let me tell you, if I could have stayed pregnant forever, it would have been just fine.

The funny thing is, I almost was pregnant forever, or so it seemed! I was ten months pregnant with no sign of labor in sight. My son was delivered by C-section because the doctor felt my son had grown too big for me to deliver him naturally.

Three months after he was born, something very strange happened: a feeling of extreme anxiety washed over me and lasted eighteen long months. My doctors said it was postpartum depression; whatever it was, it was horrific for a new, young mother to experience. Doctors had many theories: "You really do not want to be married." "You don't like motherhood." "You just aren't ready for responsibility." Let me tell you, none of that was true. I loved my son, I loved being married, and I loved the responsibility of it all!

After almost giving up, I went to see the family doctor who had taken care of me in my childhood years. I told him everything I was feeling and everything I was being told by numerous doctors. He listened and said, "I think I know what is wrong with you. Your hormones are out of balance more than they should be. Something is causing this, but I don't know what."

He sent me to Georgia to see a reproductive endocrinologist, who immediately determined I needed a hormone subcutaneous pellet to bring me back from the abyss. Every six months for twenty years, I made the trip to Georgia to get the hormone. I needed to feel better. But I was never "completely" better. It was the kind of better that gave me enough energy to take care of my family and do all the things my children needed in their growing-up years.

When I reached my perimenopausal years, I began having pain in my lower abdomen. After five years, it was finally discovered that I had endometriosis and a twisted uterus that happened after my third C-section. I had to undergo an emergency hysterectomy.

During these busy years of raising my children, taking care of a home, and tending to homework, sports, and carpools, I had been slowly losing ground. I was getting very tired, getting very stiff in my muscles, and losing my desire to go and do the things that used to bring me joy. I was wired and tired. I was gaining weight, and I was cold. My skin was very dry, and panic attacks started.

When those started, my life as I once knew it stopped.

It was then that a physician's assistant listened to me and said, "I think you may have a thyroid issue." She thought it was time to test further. She tested my thyroid antibodies and called me with the results.

"Congratulations!" she said. "You have Hashimoto's. Now we know what is going on with you."

Oh no, they didn't! Thyroid medication alone will not treat Hashimoto's. But back then, doctors did not focus on the autoimmune component. Menopause had happened for me at age thirty-eight as a result of my hysterectomy. The diagnosis of Hashimoto's came at age fifty, and it was just that—a diagnosis. With no estrogen, no progesterone, faltering thyroid levels, and exhausted adrenals, life was no fun.

Menopause and Those Pesky Hormones

What I have learned from painful experience is the delicate dance of the hormones. If you are lacking in one, all the others will suffer. You must take a holistic approach in your perimenopausal and menopausal years. If you add autoimmune thyroid disease to the mix, you have a lot to do to regain your vitality and your life.

In the years following my diagnosis of Hashimoto's, my doctors thought my symptoms were due to surgically induced menopause. They were partially right. But I was on bioidentical hormone replacement and still felt unwell. Again, the stress card came up. After all, I had a large family, a career that kept me very busy, and I was an A-type personality.

What I know now is that since Hashimoto's disease is

an immune system disease, where your immune system launches an attack on your thyroid, it takes more than a thyroid pill to make you feel well again.

Oh, and that eighteen months of hormonal hades I journeyed through as a new mom? It was my thyroid disease trying to make itself known. It often does that during the postpartum period. And that feeling of well-being during my pregnancies that I wished would last forever? Like I mentioned, high levels of progesterone contributed to that euphoria, but that increase in progesterone also helped support my thyroid function. And what about that hysterectomy because of endometriosis? That was caused by estrogen dominance and a progesterone deficiency. Progesterone facilitates thyroid function!

The takeaway from my story is to *think thyroid*—even if your TSH is normal—when you feel unwell and your symptoms keep piling up. *Think thyroid* if your body temperature is low. That is your body's cry for help. *Think thyroid* when doctors tell you everything is fine and yet you feel tired, have gained weight, have anxiety, have foggy thinking, and cannot handle stress. *Think thyroid* if your menopausal symptoms are more intense than your friends' are. If your doctor is coming up short on answers and you are long in symptoms, tell him to *think thyroid*!

Hypothyroidism's Mirror of Menopause

As you age, your endocrine system goes through changes as you progress through the stages of life. When you experience menopause, you experience a major shift in the activity of your endocrine system as some hormones decrease and the body tries to adjust. The symptoms of menopause and hypothyroidism are so similar that they can be mistaken for each other. When you reach out for help balancing menopausal hormone issues, it is important to look for hypothyroidism separately. In addition, autoimmune disease (including autoimmune hypothyroidism) has a much higher incidence of rearing its ugly head as we age, so it is important to have your thyroid carefully tested while you are supporting and balancing your sex hormone issues during this phase of your life.

Symptoms ranging from vaginal dryness and irritation to repeated miscarriages and infertility have been shown to be related to the thyroid. For many women, especially thyroid disease sufferers, menopause is treated as an illness. In actuality it is a natural passage into what I call your "wise woman" years. If you arrive with an undiagnosed and untreated thyroid disease, it can sure feel like illness as your body tries to transition into years of freedom where you no longer bear children but give birth to the dreams you have put on hold for many years. I liken this to your thyroid saying, "This is a stickup! Until you give me the thyroid hormones I need, you're not going anywhere! Literally!"

As a woman your quality of life depends on knowing the symptoms and indicators of hypothyroidism. This is especially true if you are experiencing the symptoms of menopause. Tell your doctor if you suspect that any of your symptoms might be related to thyroid function. You may have to PUSH if your therapy doesn't seem to be treating your symptoms. This is the time to insist on having thyroid blood work done, including the test for TSH and thyroid antibodies (TPO and TgAb). These simple blood tests can definitely indicate either autoimmune thyroid disease (Hashimoto's) or hypothyroidism, both of which will be treated with thyroid hormone replacement medication and dietary changes. Do not let these tests be omitted, because a clear diagnosis and treatment can make a world of difference to your current and future state of health.

Another great reason to get these tests is the fact that if you are menopausal, menopause will make your hypothyroid symptoms worse. Women who are thyroid patients have more difficulty in menopause than non-thyroid patients.

Take a look at the symptoms of both hypothyroidism and menopause. Many of the symptoms overlap. If you are having an especially hard transition from perimenopause to menopause, have your thyroid checked!

Hypothyroidism symptoms

- Fatigue
- Weight gain
- Aches and pains in joints and muscles
- Constipation
- Dry and itchy skin
- Brittle hair
- Hair loss, including loss of eyebrow hair
- Feeling cold even in warm temperatures
- Milky discharge from breasts
- Infertility
- Heavy menstrual periods
- Depression
- Mental sluggishness
- Forgetfulness
- Increased sleepiness

- Emotional instability
- Inability to focus and pay attention
- Irritability

Menopause symptoms

- Hot flashes and night sweats
- Irregular periods leading to complete cessation
- Loss of libido
- Vaginal dryness
- Difficulty concentrating; memory lapses
- Mood swings
- Fatigue
- Hair loss
- Sleep disorders; insomnia
- Dizziness
- Weight gain around the midsection
- Incontinence; bladder infection
- Anxiety, panic disorder, depression, and irritability
- Bloating, allergies
- Brittle nails
- Changes in body odor
- Irregular heartbeat and palpitations
- Breast pain and tenderness

- Headaches; migraines
- Joint pain; muscle tension
- Burning tongue; gum problems
- Electric shocks and tingling extremities
- Digestive problems
- Itchy, dry skin; rashes
- Osteoporosis

When menopause officially arrives, menstrual cycles cease and estrogen levels plummet. Since estrogen has far-reaching effects, as your other endocrine hormones do, your body will certainly alert you to the fact that you are running on empty in terms of energy. Again, even though these symptoms are clear symptoms of menopause, *always* have your thyroid checked. A properly functioning thyroid and good adrenal function will help you to move smoothly through the turbulent waters of menopause.

While symptoms of menopause and thyroid disease overlap, there are also distinct differences that you should know. In both menopause and thyroid disease you feel achy, but in different ways. Menopausal women typically have muscle tension, joint pain, and breast tenderness, whereas thyroid disease normally affects your limbs and neck by causing them to swell. (I can remember my legs feeling heavy. When I walked, it felt as though I was trudging through oatmeal.) Thyroid disease can result in loss of hair in your eyelashes or eyebrows (if I see a woman missing the outer third of her eyebrows, I ask her if she has a thyroid issue; if she says, "No," you had better believe that I tell her to have that gland checked ASAP), whereas menopause is more likely to cause the thinning of your hair on your head due to lower estrogen levels.

Weight gain is common to both hypothyroidism and menopause, as is fatigue. In the context of menopause, fatigue is a state of exhaustion that feels like your life force is being drained out of you. You are tired even after you have slept, and you are weak even after resting. This lack of energy is alarming because it seems to have no cause. It is one of the most common reasons women go to the doctor, and it is a primary menopausal symptom. You may also find yourself uncharacteristically irritable and unable to concentrate. Often these symptoms are accompanied by a crash, fatigue that occurs suddenly and leaves you without energy to function.

Many women are surprised to know that these problems are usually hormonal. Experiencing a lowered energy level and a persistent feeling of weakness or tiredness is one of the most common symptoms caused by hormonal changes. Estrogen is the primary component involved in energy levels, and when this hormone drops, especially during menopause, the energy loss is dramatic. When this hormone drops, in essence, so do you! What to do? Find a health-care provider that is schooled in bioidentical hormone replacement. By replacing your estrogen and testosterone to more youthful levels, you will feel like you have "turned back the clock." I consider bioidentical hormone replacement to be safe, as it is not synthetic and is tailored specifically to your individual hormone levels. I have been receiving bioidentical hormone replacement for almost thirty-seven years.

Now you know the similarities, so here are the differences. The weight gain and water retention of hypothyroidism occur because of insufficient amounts of thyroid hormone. This can slow down your metabolism, and with it, the way your body processes fats, proteins, and carbohydrates. The weight gain that occurs in menopause is due to the hormonal changes (lowered estrogen and testosterone) that can result in increased body fat accumulation.

One last interesting note before we move on—to further demonstrate that patients need to PUSH to find real causes for their complaints, a major medical association conducted a survey of women who were patients of their member doctors. They found that millions of the women they were treating for menopause-like symptoms, including those taking estrogen, were probably also suffering from undiagnosed thyroid disease. During the survey, The American Association of Clinical Endocrinologists (AACE) found that only one in four women who mentioned menopause-like symptoms to their doctors were tested for thyroid disease.[1] These specialists certainly know that fatigue, depression, mood swings, and sleep disturbances are key indicators of hypothyroidism but become less obvious when associated with menopause.

From the cradle to the grave, women are at the mercy of their hormones. My goal here is to educate you enough so that you will not be at the mercy of a doctor who does not pay close attention to you, your symptoms, or to the thyroid gland when it has gone awry.

Becoming pregnant, carrying a baby to term, and giving birth to a healthy child are some of the greatest joys of womanhood. Bringing a new life into the world gives a woman a joyful and tangible taste of the "circle of life." Unfortunately there is a condition that can rob a new mother of this unspeakable joy. Women worldwide, approximately one in twelve, experience the condition known as postpartum thyroiditis, which is often diagnosed as postpartum depression without even considering that a struggling, sputtering thyroid may be the root cause. The symptoms can range from periods that resemble hyperthyroidism, with anxiety, heart palpitations, and insomnia, to periods of hypothyroid-like symptoms characterized by fatigue that rest does not resolve. In the research I scoured during the writing of this important section, I found that when it comes to postpartum thyroiditis, the hyperthyroid phase typically lasts anywhere from two to six months, and then the hypothyroid phase sets in for typically three to twelve months, with a return to feeling normal around the time the baby turns one year old.[2]

I can tell you that I suffered from what was called postpartum depression for eighteen months in 1978, after the birth of my first child. I told my doctor that I really did not feel depressed! I felt anxious, had panicky feelings, could not sleep, and could hardly swallow a glass of water for fear of choking (of course, swallowing food was twice as hard). At the time doctors all agreed with the diagnosis of postpartum depression—after all, I was young, I'd had a baby right away without time to really settle into my marriage, and maybe I didn't really want to be a mother; therefore, I was depressed. *Wrong*!

I now know that I had a classic case of postpartum thyroiditis coupled with undiagnosed Hashimoto's disease. How I wish that I could have been diagnosed then instead of decades later. When I think of all of the years that my poor thyroid health was responsible for days and nights of unexplainable symptoms and frustration, tears well up in my eyes.

If you have ever experienced postpartum depression, or if your own daughter or friend is experiencing wild, life-disrupting symptoms after giving birth that seem to last for months, I encourage you (or your daughter or friend) to get your thyroid checked. Let's get you to diagnosis in days instead of decades.

MANAGING MENOPAUSE

If you are a woman who has been diagnosed as menopausal and you are being treated with estrogen, it is beyond frustrating to have no relief from your symptoms. You may even have to try to convince your doctor that you still have hot flashes, irritability, insomnia, and heart palpitations when your estrogen levels appear just fine to him after he treated you with estrogen replacement. Despite dealing with "fuzzy thinking," you can still think clearly enough to know that something else must be going on. PUSH! Once again, more often than not, treatment with the right thyroid hormone medication can not only save your sanity, but also can save your life!

When underlying hypothyroidism is treated properly, many other problems are solved as well. The thyroid gland controls many functions in your body. When it malfunctions, it causes all of your body functions to operate at a deficit. When the thyroid functions properly, many troublesome issues and symptoms literally melt away. If you are menopausal, you will still be menopausal, but it will be a much kinder and gentler process when your thyroid isn't misbehaving and causing a multitude of life-disrupting issues.

By now you have learned that your thyroid is a major player during each and every passage of your life. The level of thyroid hormone in your body will determine how well you sleep, how much energy you have, how much stamina you have, and how disrupting and severe your hot flashes will be. If your thyroid hormone level is too low, your energy goes down and your symptoms go up, your ability to handle stress is hampered, and you are less emotionally equipped to cope with all of life's challenges that normally occur during the menopausal years.

Your thyroid plays a very important part in the hormonal symphony that makes your body dance, move, and live life fully. You must be proactive and have all of your hormone levels tested during this very important time in life.

The menopausal years can be wonderful. They are the years to get back to you! It is the season of life for you to take that trip around the world, write that book, take that class, buy that boat and sail it, and fall in love again. It is the time to cherish all that you were, all that you are, and all that you are going to be from now on. And all of these things can be done with much more joy if your hormones are balanced and an underlying thyroid condition is addressed.

Chapter 11

FINDING (HORMONE) BALANCE

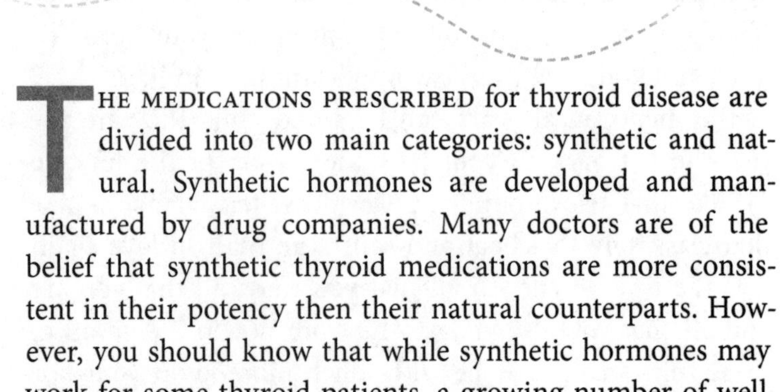

THE MEDICATIONS PRESCRIBED for thyroid disease are divided into two main categories: synthetic and natural. Synthetic hormones are developed and manufactured by drug companies. Many doctors are of the belief that synthetic thyroid medications are more consistent in their potency then their natural counterparts. However, you should know that while synthetic hormones may work for some thyroid patients, a growing number of well-educated thyroid patients realize the important difference between synthetic and natural hormone replacement, and have made the switch to a more natural treatment. Synthetic thyroid hormone medications contain T4 alone, T3, or both; their brand names are Synthroid, Levothroid, Levoxyl, Unithroid, Cytomel, and Thyrolar.

Prescription medications that fall into the natural category consist of hormone tissue that is extracted from beef or hog thyroids. These naturally derived thyroid medications so closely resemble what your thyroid normally produces that your body readily accepts them. These hormone replacements, known as desiccated thyroid hormones, are produced under the brand names Armour, Nature-Throid, and Westhroid.

During your thyroid recovery journey, you will no doubt come across endocrinologists who insist you take synthetic versus natural thyroid hormone medications. The majority of doctors and endocrinologists have been convinced by the drug companies that their synthetic products are scientifically more reliable and accurate. A growing number of doctors are now open to natural desiccated hormones (NDTs) and will recommend the kind of hormone that is more effective for each patient. Many patients have tried a variety of medications, and a large percentage find that they prefer the natural thyroid hormone replacement over the synthetic brands. Keep in mind that natural thyroid hormones were in use way before the synthetic medications were developed. I have found natural thyroid hormones very effective at keeping my thyroid hormone levels consistent, as have my daughters.

If your blood work points to a straightforward case of hypothyroidism, your next move is to begin thyroid hormone replacement therapy. It may take some time to find what thyroid medication works best for your particular system. Some people do well on T4 only (like Synthroid), which I will discuss more below.

Please note that T4-only therapy may be problematic for many people. The body must convert that T4 into active T3, which the body uses for energy, and many people have a hard time converting T4 into T3. The physician may "dose up" in order to bring your blood levels into normal range, when all the while the problem lies in the conversion. Sadly many patients go years without optimal treatment.

An exception to the rule is the group of patients who find they actually do feel better on synthetic hormone replacement such as Synthroid. These patients typically have Hashimoto's, and their bodies are producing antibodies to their own thyroid tissue and their own thyroid hormones. When these patients are given desiccated thyroid hormone replacement such as Armour, it causes their bodies to produce antibodies to the natural thyroid medication because it is so similar to their own thyroid tissue, and their symptoms get worse as a result. In this case the thyroid does not produce antibodies to the synthetic medication, so it becomes the more effective solution for this special group of autoimmune thyroid disease sufferers.

Still, for the majority of patients, desiccated thyroid hormone is what can make all the difference. It can be life changing. Desiccated thyroid hormone contains not only T4 but also T1, T2, and T3. This makes it more physiologically compatible, and it does not make your body work hard to convert it.

How well you feel will help to determine which thyroid hormone works the best in your particular case. Make sure you find a doctor who treats more than the blood work. Seek out a doctor who treats the patient—that's you. This is a huge factor. Blood work alone will not tell the entire story. This is especially true when dealing with autoimmune thyroid disease.

THE THIRD CUT IS THE DEEPEST

When you are dealing with a thyroid disease such as Hashimoto's or hypothyroidism, you will gain weight and have a hard time losing it. Any hypothyroid condition will slow down your metabolic rate. In my case, I gained twenty-five to thirty pounds and was devastated about it. I tried everything I knew to do, but the excess poundage would not budge. I did not realize that autoimmune thyroid disease was affecting my ability to shed the unwanted pounds.

What I have learned is that there are three areas to take into consideration when trying to regain your proper scale digits:

1. Diet
2. Exercise
3. Hormone balance

I was very aware of the fact that diet modification was one way to lose weight. I always ate healthy foods, so I just made sure to eat early and often to keep my metabolism running smoothly. I ate ample servings of vegetables each day, plus salads and low-glycemic fruits like blueberries and strawberries. I ate leans meats like organic chicken and turkey. I ate fish, such as wild-caught salmon. But still my weight did not budge. I felt as if my entire body was rebelling against me. Little did I know, it really was.

My energy levels were getting increasingly lower, and I could no longer take my long, stress-relieving walks. I chalked it all up to stress, because the parade of health-care providers insisted that was the case.

What I didn't know at the time was that if you have Hashimoto's thyroid disease or hypothyroidism, you have a hormonal imbalance. If you have a hormonal imbalance, it will be extremely hard, if not impossible, to lose weight by simply eating right and exercising (provided you even have the energy to attempt it).

Factor #1: Diet

Diet is very important and is certainly first and foremost in any weight-loss program. In addition to eating fresh, early, and often—early in the day, not after 6:00 p.m., and six small meals daily—make sure you don't skip breakfast; otherwise your blood sugar levels will be off kilter. After eating a healthy breakfast, which should contain protein and no grains and be low glycemic, make sure to eat a small, protein-packed snack every two to three hours at the least. This will keep your blood sugar stable and will help to curb your appetite.

People with autoimmune thyroid conditions, or any thyroid issue, should eat something within an hour of waking up. Again, this serves to keep your blood sugar stable, and gives you much-needed energy to begin your day.

Given that most people with thyroid issues have adrenal issues as well, there is a tendency to use caffeine to get that jolt of energy to start the day. It is important to know that while this may work in the short run, in the long run your adrenal glands (which you are trying to support and heal) will be further taxed. So your best bet here is to slowly wean off caffeine and derive energy from eating fresh, eating early, and eating often. (Decaf coffee is permissible if you love the taste of coffee in the morning.)

Focus on lean meats and vegetables, and eliminate all grains. Completely eliminate refined foods because they can cause a spike in your blood sugar, which over the course of months or even years will put stress on your adrenal glands and pancreas. In the case of Hashimoto's or Graves' disease, the autoimmune system is involved, and it is imperative that dietary steps be taken to help control it.

Factor #2: Exercise

Once you have all of these dietary recommendations in place, you should then begin a walking program. The importance of exercise cannot be overlooked with an autoimmune disease, even though the thought of it repulses you. It feels downright insulting when well-meaning friends and family members tell you, "Just take a walk—you'll feel better." The truth is, you will not feel better unless and until you get your diagnosis and start to implement the dietary, lifestyle, and hormonal balancing support you actually need.

Once you have your diagnosis and begin to feel your

energy return, albeit slowly in most cases, you should try to walk for thirty minutes three to five days a week as an ultimate goal. Again, this will seem impossible for those that have been hit especially hard with this stealthy, devastating illness that robs you of yourself so slowly that one day, you suddenly wake up wondering where you went!

One important thing to remember here is that having undiagnosed thyroid disease, especially autoimmune thyroid disease, is often a very lonely experience. At least it was for me. I knew something was wrong, but what? What was stealing my zest for life, my joy, and all of the things that I loved to participate in? I kept my feeling of disease hidden by making excuses for not attending so many things that used to bring me great joy. People often do not understand how poorly you are feeling. They don't understand how you can feel so badly when you don't look sick. That is why thyroid disease is often called the "invisible illness."

When you start walking, with each step you take, picture yourself reclaiming your health and your life, one step at a time. This is not a marathon by society's standards. It is a personal *camino*, a walk from the dark days of illness into the light of understanding how to manage it and regain life. It is a very personal comeback.

Along the way, you will have feelings arise that need to be processed and purged. Something I personally had to do was forgive all of the misdiagnoses and negligence when it came to health-care providers not listening to my symptoms. It was insulting, it was stressful, it was devastating, and it was expensive, both financially and spiritually.

Another factor to consider when you are trying to shed weight is shedding harmful emotions. In my many nights of research into this formidable foe, I read over and over that thyroid problems are the result of a stagnation in the throat area as a result of not expressing oneself—in other words, holding back or not saying what you really think or feel. In my case I am sure this was true on some level, as I lived for many years with the disease to please and did not express my true feelings or take action to correct things in my life that were eating me up inside.

One thing I know for sure here is that after dealing with it all, I now speak my truth, and I don't hold back because of any fear I may have of expressing myself. I will never do that again.

Factor #3: Hormones

Now we come to the hormone component of weight loss. Again, if you have a thyroid condition, you have a hormonal imbalance. This makes it very hard to lose weight just by exercising and eating right. This is where imbalances of cortisol, thyroid hormones, and insulin, as well as estrogen dominance, come into play. You must seek out a functional medicine physician who can test your levels by running a hormonal assay.

When your hormones are properly balanced, weight loss happens, especially when you also pay attention to your diet and exercise regimen. This is not to be taken lightly if you want to get back to the real you—the person that you and your family recognize. Doing these things will not only help you get back to the weight you were before the thyroid madness all began, but it will help you keep it off for good. It will also help to keep the rest of your system healthy and functioning up to par.

In addition to taking optimal doses of thyroid hormone medication, you will need:

- Digestive enzymes
- Probiotics

- Curcumin
- Resveratrol
- Vitamin D

Be sure to have your adrenal glands checked before you begin taking thyroid medication. Why? Because starting thyroid meds with weak adrenal glands can cause you to feel much worse. Many aware physicians know to make sure the adrenals are strong enough to handle the addition of thyroid hormone. If they are not up to snuff, then the adrenals should be supported simultaneously with licorice root, ashwagandha, pantothenic acid, or, in severe cases, physiological doses of hydrocortisone four times a day. My daughters and I had almost no cortisol, and my younger daughter and I had a hard time utilizing thyroid hormone after our thyroidectomies, so we had to resort to supporting our adrenal glands with the hormones that were so depleted (hydrocortisone).

Addison's disease is an autoimmune disease of the adrenal glands. Starting a person on thyroid hormones without testing for Addison's is, in my opinion, risky. My daughters and I were two points away from being diagnosed with Addison's. I pushed until doctors agreed that we did in fact need physiological dosing of cortisol since our adrenals had almost no output. Believe it or not, all thyroid medication package inserts state that thyroid hormone should never be given to a person with undiagnosed, untreated, or poorly managed adrenal disease. To do so can be dangerous.

To summarize, you must focus on diet, exercise, and optimal hormonal balance, not just thyroid hormone. Having thyroid disease creates deficits in the other endocrine hormones, so it is very important to make sure that your levels are all optimal.

Chapter 12

THE THYROID AND THE GUT

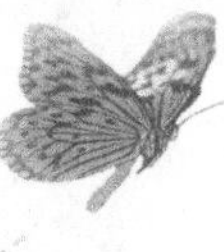

LEAKY GUT HAS been found to be a major causative factor in autoimmune disease. Eighty percent of your immunity resides in your gut. Years of antibiotic use, steroids, NSAIDS, processed foods, sugar, yeast overgrowth, and stress can cause inflammation that results in holes in the cell junctions that make up your gut. Once this happens, toxins can enter your bloodstream. Your body sees these toxins as invaders and begins to seek and destroy. The problem is that it is *you* that your body starts to destroy. There are over eighty known autoimmune diseases, and evidence points to all of them beginning with inflammation in the gut.

My daughters and I had taken many antibiotics during our lives. The trouble is, antibiotics kill all the good bacteria as well as the bad in the gut, and thus contribute to yeast overgrowth by killing and crowding out healthy intestinal flora (probiotics or good bacteria). Yeast overgrowth is dependent on sugar for its proliferation, so it causes a craving for sugar, carbohydrates, and starches. The more you feed the yeast beast, the more it grows, sending symptoms to every system of your body.

We had headaches, joint pain, allergies, shortness of breath, and anxiety. Even though we all took vitamins, herbs, and minerals—even detoxification cleanses—we still had issues. All of this was happening during my daughters' busy "growing years," when school projects, activities, carpooling, and the business of family life kept our eyes off the ball that was snowballing toward something that would be devastating to our health in years to come. Our diet was rich in grains, pasta, and wheat bread.

Little did we know that our guts' integrity was being compromised by the inflammation that would soon create leaky gut. Once you have a leaky gut, everything you eat becomes a potential antigen or a perceived invader for your immune system to wage war against—an unseen war within that rages twenty-four hours a day.

The Breast Is Best

I'm going to begin our discussion of leaky gut in a place you wouldn't expect—by telling you that from the moment of my birth, the stage was set for autoimmunity. I mentioned in chapter 1 that I was not breast-fed and was born prematurely. These two factors, along with a genetic predisposition for autoimmune disease and a childhood and young adulthood filled with illness and trauma, were my triggers.

William Parker, PhD, associate professor of surgery at Duke University School of Medicine, sums up the importance of breast milk in the autoimmunity challenge. He says:

> Research in my lab at Duke has shown very large differences between breast milk and baby formulas in terms of how they help a baby's healthy, necessary bacteria grow. Simply put, if you mix normal bacteria with breast milk in a test tube, the bacteria do the normal things that they would do in your baby. If you mix the same exact bacteria with baby formula in a test tube, the bacteria grow in a completely different way. The normal mode of bacterial growth in the gut is to form protective films of living bacteria we call "biofilms." Mother's milk helps this happen. Infant formulas, on

> the other hand, induce the bacteria into prolific growth as single, free-floating cells. The bacteria grow very fast, but they remain nomadic and don't stick together. The difference is huge and can easily be seen in a test tube with a simple experiment. Infant formulas are just not the same as mother's milk in terms of how they affect healthy bacterial growth.
>
> We know that the development of our baby's immune system is dependent on the friendly bacteria in our baby, and now we know how much the normal growth of this friendly bacteria depends on breast milk. With this in mind, it seems more than worthwhile to avoid yet another risk factor. It pays to give our babies breast milk.
>
> Human milk is awash in secretory IgA (sIgA), an antibody that floods the newborn's mucous membranes (gut, lungs, etc.), helps build the healthy biofilm, and acts as the first line of defense in fighting infection and disease.[1]

Interestingly enough, research has shown that babies born by cesarean section have a greater risk of developing a host of illnesses as well. Researchers have found distinct differences in the type of bacteria in the intestinal tracts of babies that were delivered by C-section compared to those who had a vaginal birth. The researchers have concluded that these microbial differences could have lifelong health consequences for children, such as chronic inflammation, autoimmunity, allergies, and chronic illness.[2]

Here is why. The adult human gut is teeming with billions of "friendly" bacteria that aid digestion and help guard against pathogens, but a newborn's belly is virtually devoid of microbes. Normally a child's first exposure to bacteria occurs during the passage down the mother's vaginal canal. The infant becomes covered in bacteria, and some is ingested. The infant picks up more bacteria from mom through breast-feeding. In this fashion the child's gut becomes populated with beneficial bacteria that also play a critical role in developing the infant's immune system.

However, a child who is delivered by C-section essentially bypasses this initial bacterial dunking. What's more, women who have C-sections tend to delay breast-feeding, and they are given antibiotics to ward off infections in their incisions—proof again that autoimmunity does begin in the gut.

Would it surprise you to learn that both my daughters—who have both battled severe symptoms of Hashimoto's disease and the youngest of whom lost her thyroid to papillary thyroid cancer—were born by cesarean section? Without that healthy gut bacteria from a vaginal birth, they both started life compromised.

My theory is that those genes that trigger autoimmunity are likely more easily expressed (turned "on") when gut flora is poor. In my case I was not breast-fed and had a hard time keeping formula down. As a result I was sickly and lived on antibiotics for most of my childhood. Both of my daughters were delivered by C-section. My oldest daughter was breast-fed but suffered from allergies as a child, and my youngest, who almost died at birth, lost her urge to nurse. Note that my youngest was born by C-section and was not breast-fed, and it is my youngest who has suffered the most.

What did all three of us have in common? Poor gut flora. I believe that was our main trigger, along with genetic predisposition. Again, I do not believe the genes for autoimmunity would have had to express if our emergence from our mothers' womb had been ideal.

Genetics are responsible for 25 percent of the risk of developing an autoimmune disease; 75 percent is environmental or can be chalked up to epigenetics, meaning the risks you are exposed to in your lifetime.

EPIGENETICS: THE NEW TRIGGER

The concept of genetics is that we are born with innate characteristics that cannot be changed. Today that position has changed. Geneticists now tell us that external factors can alter genes and create new patterns of susceptibility to disease that didn't exist at birth. This field of science is called epigenetics, which means "above genetics." The new findings show that factors such as trauma, diet, stress, exposure to toxins, and childbirth can imprint genes with conditions a person was not hardwired for by his or her parents' DNA.

While some forms of stress create a harmful genetic profile, other forms of stress actually go to the good. This kind of stress is identified by the term *eustress*. Natural childbirth is understood to be a producer of eustress that promotes a healthy and positive outcome on the fetus. On the other hand, a birth by cesarean section does not provide eustress. It has been proven that the child delivered by C-section has a greater disposition for type 1 diabetes, asthma and allergies, autoimmune disorders, gastroenteritis, obesity, eczema, and some forms of cancer.[3]

When genes are impressed with eustress during natural labor and birth, the resulting genetic changes are called the epigenomic effect. This term defines the reprogramming or remodeling that takes place in the genes. We now know that the birth process and labor chemistry establish programming for either a normal or abnormal gene expression that will manifest later in life. These results can play a major role in shaping our immunity, weight regulation, tumor suppression, and even behavioral problems. Epigenetics suggests that your life will take on patterns not only from your parents but also from how you were born.

The Balancing Act

Remember that all autoimmunity begins in the gut. Yes, genetic predisposition is involved. But genes do not have to express. Triggers instigate the autoimmune disease process. Stress is a huge trigger in the autoimmunity cascade that contributes to adrenal exhaustion. In addition, overuse of antibiotics can disrupt healthy intestinal flora, as can a poor diet with too many refined and sugary foods, fried foods, and caffeine. This leads to leaky gut. Leaky gut, as you have learned, sets the stage for systemic inflammation. Inflammation, if not addressed, is fertile ground from which autoimmunity springs forth.

I have always told my clients, "If you don't feel well, go with your gut!" Most of your immune system resides in your gut, so it is easy to understand why I always stress the importance of beginning your journey back to health by fixing what I call "the cradle of immunity," the gut.

Your gut is teeming with bacteria, both good and bad. The good bacteria should ideally make up 80 to 85 percent, and the bad bacteria should make up only 15 to 20 percent. When your gut bacteria is in this ideal range, you will feel strong and well, with few if any cold and flu infections, good disease-fighting antibody levels, and regular elimination. Your digestion will not be an issue, and your body will easily absorb vitamins and nutrients from your foods.

Conversely, when your gut bacteria is populated with more of the bad bacteria than good, the stage is set for a myriad of health complaints including gut inflammation and/or infection, constipation, diarrhea, candida yeast infections, food allergies, headaches, leaky gut, and lowered immunity. All of these issues set the stage for autoimmunity.

The biggest disrupters of a healthy gut bacteria ratio are antibiotics, antacids, and stress. The first two issues can be rectified by taking a daily probiotic to replace the healthy bacteria that were wiped out by the medications. Stress, however, is a fact of life, so you must learn to not let it destroy your health. Remember, it is easier to maintain your health than to try to regain it! Learn to not sweat the small stuff. If you become ill, you will soon learn that everything else that you once worried about suddenly becomes small stuff.

TAKING CARE OF YOUR GUT

Gut health tip #1

Eliminate gluten to help stop inflammation, and take a probiotic supplement each and every day to help keep your gut ratio of good bacteria where it needs to be for optimal health. This is especially true if you have taken long or repeated courses of antibiotics throughout your lifetime. It has recently come to light that persons who were not breastfed as infants and/or who were delivered by C-section live their lives compromised in terms of good, disease-fighting gut bacteria that is normally bestowed upon us by way of the birth canal, breast milk, or both. If this is true in your case, a probiotic is essential! Medications such as steroids and antacids wreak havoc on your gut bacteria ratio, as well as a diet laden with sugary, fried, artificially flavored, and refined foods.

In addition to taking a daily probiotic, I recommend that you take a digestive enzyme from a plant source to help you assimilate and digest your food with ease. When it comes to healing the body from autoimmune thyroid disease, the goal is to take the load off the immune system and get the inflammation down.

Keeping your gut wall amply covered with good bacteria is your body's first line of defense since the day you took your first breath. It is now your job to keep it covered.

Gut health tip #2

Eat whole foods. If it doesn't rot or sprout, do without! Eat as close to the original garden as possible, and add fermented foods that are chock full of good bacteria, like sauerkraut, kefir, kimchi, and miso. Adding garlic, onions, artichokes, and bananas to your diet will act as prebiotics, which act as food for probiotics, thereby enhancing their growth.

Gut health tip #3

Another very important way to support your gut health is to stay hydrated. Your gut depends on water to keep inflammation down and to keep bacteria and wastes moving through your system all the way to elimination. That is way we call it a bowel *movement*. To ensure that you are adequately hydrated, simply take your current weight and divide by two. Your answer will be the number of ounces of water you need daily to keep your body afloat, so to speak, with all systems "go!"

Gut health tip #4

Avoid refined sugar and processed foods. This one is easy. Bad bacteria *love* sugar! One way to keep the bad bacteria population down, which also includes resultant yeast overgrowth, is to simply avoid sugar and processed foods. Focus on eating plant-based, whole foods that are nutrient dense.

Gut health tip #5

Your gut has a brain. When it comes to healing, there is a big connection between your gut and your brain. What affects your gut, affects your brain, and vice versa. Your gut is often referred to as "your second brain."

How many times have you had a "gut feeling" about something stressful? It is interesting to note that there are receptors in your gut that are identical to the ones in your brain. When you are faced with a stressful situation, your brain and gut react together. But you will feel it more profoundly in the gut, because stress causes your digestion, blood flow, and muscles in the gut to slow way down. You will feel this as indigestion, constipation, bloating, and gas pain.

Finally, to take the very best care of your gut and brain, you must learn to cope with stress. Try deep breathing, prayer, meditation, massage therapy, uplifting relationships, and quiet walks in the outdoors.

Chapter 13

AGAINST THE GRAIN

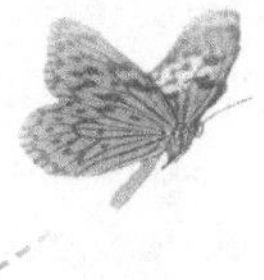

In terms of thyroid disease, especially autoimmune disease, the connection to wheat gluten—especially to our "new wheat"—is very strong. Here is a clear breakdown of GMO wheat and the ramifications of consuming it.

It is reported that 80 to 90 percent of today's commercial food crops such as corn, wheat, and soy are GMOs. Everyone has heard the term *GMO* by now and that we should probably stay away from them for health reasons. But few people know exactly what GMOs are. Here is your primer. GMO stands for "genetically modified organism." How are organisms genetically modified? Plants and animals can be genetically modified in a lab by combining the DNA of different species by cross breeding or other methods not found in nature.

It makes sense that to date, we do not know the long-term effects of consuming GMO foods, although preliminary evidence is pointing to a potential link to autoimmunity. Therefore it is my personal belief that you should avoid all GMO foods. I read labels, I read the research, and you should too! Read all that you can, because your health and the health of your children and children's children may depend on it. I feel this is especially true if you have been diagnosed with autoimmune thyroid disease, since there is a strong link to wheat gluten, and the chances of the wheat gluten being GMO or "new wheat" is very high. You should know that since their introduction in the United States in 1996, there has been a whopping 100 percent increase in persons who suffer from three or more chronic illnesses![1]

Thankfully progress is now being made in terms of requiring all GMO products to make themselves known to the consumer by clearly labeling them as such. That is the good news. The not so good news is that until then, you probably don't even know when you're eating GMO food in many cases. Back to the good news—there are some ways to avoid these potentially problematic foods that can rob you of your health and ability to live life to the fullest.

Here is a list of the most common GMO foods:

1. Soy
2. Corn (including high-fructose corn syrup, corn oil, and corn syrup)
3. Canola oil
4. Cotton (including cottonseed oil)
5. Milk
6. Sugar
7. Aspartame
8. Zucchini
9. Yellow squash
10. Papaya[2]

Why You Should Avoid GMOs

The following information will probably go against the grain of the giant companies that produce GMO food, but I feel it is my duty to share what I have found to be true. I no longer ingest *any* grains due to my development of autoimmunity. I am doing all that I can to quell inflammation and heal my leaky gut now and for the rest of my life. My children are doing the same. When you have been dealt the wild card of autoimmunity in any area of your body, your goal is to do all that you can to get to the root cause. Healing the gut is imperative. Getting the oh-so-inflammatory GMO grains out of your life can make a world of difference, and a difference to your world.

Here Are the Facts

1. GMOs have increased the use of herbicides.

One of the main selling points of genetic engineering is the creation of more pest-resistant crops. The downside is that chemical- and pest-resistant weeds now infest farmers' fields. This has resulted in the development of "superweeds" that have required farmers to resort to using more and more herbicides to kill them. But these resistant weeds are still growing and spreading. These dangerous chemicals are used in higher and higher amounts as an antidote to increased resistance, eventually making their way into your body via the food you eat. I liken this to what occurs when you take too many antibiotics. Too many antibiotics leads to more and more antibiotic-resistant infections. Bigger and bigger "antibiotic guns" are then used to knock out the superbugs, which in turn knock out your immunity. In the same way, the heavier doses of herbicides ultimately take a heavy toll on your health.

2. It is poorly understood that GMO's have disease-causing potential.

At the present time the research about the safety of GMOs is left up to the manufacturer. In addition there is no requirement that I could find requiring the safety of GMOs to be guaranteed. Something to consider: if profit is the driving force behind huge corporations, why would a company that is *the* biggest producer of genetically modified seeds (Monsanto) want to acknowledge that their products promote chronic disease, even in the face of emerging studies?

If rats fed a diet of GMO corn suffered increased tumor growth and early death when compared to a control group, and similar studies on GMO animal feed prompted the American Academy of Environmental Medicine (AAEM) to publicly denounce GMOs in the food supply, stating that "it is biologically plausible for Genetically Modified Foods to cause adverse health effects in humans,"[3] then why wouldn't the huge manufacturer of GMOs stop their sales? The answer is clear: profits over people! GMOs have been associated with a long list of health problems, including thyroid cancer, kidney disease, rheumatoid arthritis (which I was diagnosed with at the same time as my thyroid cancer), and infertility.[4] Is this evidence convincing to me? You bet it is!

What's done is done, and I don't think we will ever go back. Listen to this bit of information. Today's GMO crops are altered to make them resistant to both weather and pests. Corn has been engineered to produce a natural insecticide known as Bt toxin, which we in turn ultimately ingest. This toxin was developed to kill insects by destroying the cell walls of their digestive tract.[5] It is interesting to note that Bt toxin has also been shown to injure or destroy the cells that line our intestines, which in turn causes leaky gut. In other words, this toxin not only destroys an insect's digestive tract, but it also destroys ours over time. What's more, this potent chemical cannot be washed or scrubbed off because it's part of the physical structure of GMO corn.[6]

3. GMOs cross-contaminate non-GMO crops.

Something you should know: farmers cannot protect against cross-pollination, which happens naturally by insects and the wind. This is a frightening observation, because this means that non-GMO crops can be tainted—or contaminated, if you will—by this natural process, thus creating a "hybrid" of a non-GMO crop and a GMO crop. This means that the chances of finding a true non-GMO crop are not good, and there is really not much that can be done to halt it.

Since we really don't know *all* of the ramifications of eating GMO food (and signs are telling us there are many), this could be disastrous.

Two Practical Ways to Avoid GMOs

1. Buy organic—be wise!

Look for labels that say "100 percent organic" or "USDA Organic." This ensures that food is free of pesticides, herbicides, chemicals, and hormones, and is non-GMO. If the label states "made with organic," it may still contain GMOs. You must be a wise reader of labels.

2. Buy grass-fed meat and dairy. You are what they eat!

It is becoming more and important to pay attention to what your food eats, as your health can be affected by what the animal eats. GMOs can end up in your system even if the animal was not genetically modified.

Look for "certified grass fed and organic" on labels when buying meat. If you do not see this label, the animal was fed a diet that consisted of GMO feed. Remember, since GMO crops are less expensive because they are more plentiful, they are the first choice for most of the animal feed in the United States.

"ROUNDUP" THE GLUTEN

Now that you have learned that exposure to any type of gluten can cause an immune reaction that can be destructive to your intestines, your brain, your nervous system, and in a person with Hashimoto's, your thyroid, here is yet another reason why wheat may be toxic to your health.

You may have heard of the popular herbicide called Roundup. Roundup is Monsanto's most well-known product and has become part of their plan for total domination of the world's seed supply. What's more interesting is that Monsanto is actually gearing up to sue the state of Vermont because the Vermont legislature voted to label GMO foods.[7] Labeling GMO foods is great for us, but not so great for Monsanto!

Vermont is going to be the first state to make history by fighting to require GMO foods to be labeled as such. Monsanto, the world's largest producer of GMOs, is preparing to rise to the challenge and sue the state. With the help of a generous donation from SumOfUs (a group dedicated to fighting for people over profits), Vermont is fighting back! Vermont will not be the only state that will fight for GMO labeling; as Vermont and Monsanto go to trial, other states are joining in demanding that GMO labeling be required.[8]

Monsanto knows that this could be the beginning of other state legislatures voting yes to the labeling of GMO foods. This would greatly affect Monsanto's profits, because more and more informed consumers are boycotting GMO foods. Monsanto makes enormous profits on Roundup and all of the seeds that they have bred and patented so that many farmers are forced to buy their seeds from them.

But there is another use for Roundup that even the most aware non-GMO advocate does not know. Roundup is sprayed on wheat crops just before they are harvested! This is because it dries out and ripens the crop, making all parts of the harvest uniformly dry. This is a benefit to farmers because different sections of a wheat field normally ripen at different times. Farmers in Great Britain and the United States have been using it to help uniformly dry out and ripen their wheat fields a day or two before they begin to harvest.[9]

What this means to you and me is that we are not only getting GMOs from the seeds that are planted, grown, matured, and harvested, but we are also being exposed to Roundup-sprayed wheat. This means that Roundup is *in* our wheat and *on* our wheat.

The danger of glyphosate, the main chemical found in Roundup, is not going unnoticed. Since the spraying of glyphosate on US wheat crops started in 1990, cases of celiac disease (an autoimmune disease of the intestinal tract) have risen dramatically.[10] Europe is now realizing the dangers, and the Netherlands has completely banned the use of Roundup. France is on board as well and also recognizes the danger.[11]

The United States and the United Kingdom continue to use Roundup to uniformly dry their wheat crops for harvest, and glyphosate residue is found in bread samples. While the use of Roundup may make harvesting easier and ultimately more profitable for farmers, it can be disastrous to the health of the consumer who will eventually consume glyphosate residue in their wheat-based foods.[12]

All of the adverse health ramifications are just now rearing their ugly heads, and they are very ugly. Autoimmune disease can be not only damaging to your insides, but also disfiguring to your outside appearance.

THE EFFECTS OF "CROP SPRAYING"

New research has uncovered the destructive effects of Roundup and glyphosate on the digestive tract. These include:

- Disruption of the gut bacteria. When the gut wall is compromised by poor levels of beneficial gut bacteria, leaky gut can occur, opening the door to autoimmunity. Roundup has been shown to disrupt the gut's microbiome, which contributes to leaky gut.
- Increase in leaky gut. Since glyphosate can contribute to leaky gut, it follows that glyphosate-soaked gluten can slip through loose intestinal junctures and go directly into your bloodstream, ultimately ending up in your brain. This can cause brain fog, inflammation, allergies, pain, and autoimmunity in every part of your body.[13]

When you add up all of the dangerous implications, glyphosate and gluten should be avoided at all costs. This is especially true for those of us with Hashimoto's disease.

The link between celiac disease and autoimmune thyroid disease has been well established. A significant number of patients with autoimmune thyroid disease also have celiac disease, an autoimmune disease for which the treatment is the avoidance of all gluten. Maybe this is because celiac and autoimmune thyroid diseases like Hashimoto's share a common genetic predisposition. It has been shown that patients with autoimmune thyroid disease are four to fifteen times more likely to have celiac disease than the general population. But genes do *not* have to express themselves and cause disease. Something must trigger autoimmune diseases, including both celiac and Hashimoto's thyroid disease. Stress is a huge trigger!

But, in the context of this chapter, avoid *all* grains to help quell the pain and associated symptoms of autoimmune thyroiditis (Hashi's) and its travel companion, celiac disease, or gluten allergy.

Since autoimmune diseases often travel in pairs or even threes, let me also remind you here that if you have Hashimoto's thyroiditis, you should be screened for celiac disease. If you suffer with known celiac disease, you should be screened for Hashimoto's thyroiditis.

How to Hush Hashi's

If you have been diagnosed with Hashimoto's disease, your lifestyle needs to change. We discussed this a bit in chapter 8, but since this chapter deals with tending to Hashimoto's disease, I am now going to tell you exactly what to do.

Step 1: Eliminate gluten—permanently

> As far as the connection to gluten, there's just no question that many people that have Hashimoto's and hypothyroidism have gluten-sensitivity. For some patients, it's life-changing when they go gluten-free.[14]
>
> —Datis Kharrazian, DHSc. DC, MS

I cannot stress this enough: if you have Hashimoto's disease, you must become gluten free. If you want to have a fighting chance at turning the volume down on your condition and decreasing your antibody number, the gluten must go. I personally have chosen to eliminate all grains from my diet since they can cross-react. It has made an incredible difference! As you eliminate gluten, you will see your antibodies start to drop, which will start the process of healing your gut.

You need to eliminate sugars, cakes, pies, ice cream, and all grains, because there can be cross-reactivity. I am also going to recommend that you eliminate the most common problem foods, such as corn, soy, dairy, and eggs, to help you heal your gut sooner. You may use almond milk instead of dairy.

After three weeks you may add in dairy to see if you feel any sign of reaction, such as congestion, increased joint pain, skin breakouts, bloating, headaches, or fatigue. If you feel well after adding dairy back into your diet, then try adding eggs back in. If you react, then leave them out. Soy, on the other hand, is not recommended for anyone with thyroid disease.

It is important for you to know that even the most knowledgeable gluten-free adherents may not realize that there are things besides food that you must avoid to abide by a gluten-free life. Even handling a gluten-based product such as dog food, cosmetics, and skin lotions, and even breathing in the air at your local bakery or pizzeria can cause problems. Mamma mia!

Here is a list of several hidden or unexpected sources of gluten.

- Sunscreen
- Cosmetics, including lipsticks
- Certain vitamins and medications
- Envelopes and stamps
- Sauces for meats and salads
- Toothpaste

- Shampoo, conditioner, and soap
- Frying oils
- Shared cutting boards or utensils
- Grain-based sweeteners, such as malt or corn sugar
- Thickening agents used in processed foods
- Pickles
- Soy sauce
- Licorice
- Flavored potato chips
- Salad dressing[15]

You must be hypervigilant when it comes to reading labels. The goal here is to get all the offenders out. It will take willpower, and you must be strict, but the payoff is worth it. Once autoimmune disease has taken hold, it is a hard-to-conquer foe. It will take an all-out effort to hush Hashi's. By doing what I have suggested, you will give your overworked immune system a much-needed rest.

Step 2: Replenish

While you are holding fast to the "no gluten" lifestyle, you should be doing all that you can to help heal and restore the integrity of your gut. This is where adding a good probiotic (beneficial bacteria) to your daily routine comes into play. Look for one that has an abundance of healthy gut bacteria, such as bifidobacterium and lactobacillus. This will help to restock your "intestinal pond" with the good guys in white hats. Then it's time to add in digestive enzymes from a plant source, along with hydrochloric acid (HCl), since thyroid issues can impair your stomach's acid production.

If you have long-standing thyroid disease, or if you are discovering that what you have learned thus far describes you, take a good digestive enzyme a few minutes before each meal and HCl toward the end of your meal. Doing this will help you more completely digest your food again, which will in turn efficiently deliver more nutrients to your system. By taking digestive enzymes, you are taking yet another step toward damping down the autoimmune response.

Step 3: Renew

After committing to a gluten-free life, taking daily probiotics, and supplementing your body with HCl and digestive enzymes from a plant source, the next stop in the autoimmune defense toolbox is to commit to a new way of eating. I have decided to eat grain free and sugar free, and have been following what is called the Paleo diet, otherwise known as the "Caveman Diet." I now eat lean protein, plenty of vegetables, healthy fats, and bone broth from either chicken or beef. Of course I make sure that I source all beef and chicken to make sure that it is organic. I also make sure to drink plenty of water and limit caffeine, as it is too dehydrating.

I personally recommend the Paleo diet to help aid your recovery. It is the diet change I made to turn down the inflammation that tortured my body. See chapter 14 for complete details on my autoimmune recovery diet.

Chapter 14

THE AUTOIMMUNE RECOVERY DIET

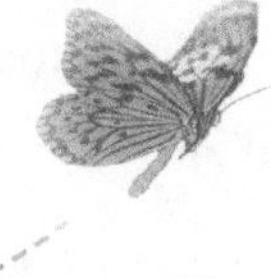

YOU'VE NOW HEARD my long story of my journey to diagnosis and recovery. Perhaps you're wondering how I stay healthy on a daily basis.

Let me tell you the specifics.

MY DAILY PROTOCOL

I no longer have a thyroid gland, so I take a thyroid medication called Nature-Throid daily. I also have mild adrenal insufficiency and must take hydrocortisone in physiological doses equivalent to 20 mg daily. (Please note that most people can support their adrenal glands by simply taking adaptogenic herbs like ashwagandha, ginseng, or licorice root, or vitamin C and pantothenic acid. It is important to have your adrenal glands' function evaluated, preferably by a naturopath or functional medicine physician, as they usually run an Adrenal Stress Index salivary cortisol test to determine just how well your adrenal glands are performing.)

I have eliminated all grains and legumes. This includes wheat, rye, barley, rice, quinoa, millet, amaranth, beans, peas, and lentils.

I have adopted a modified Paleolithic diet, otherwise known as the autoimmune protocol diet (AIP). The goal of this diet is to calm inflammation in the gut and as a result, the body. Most elimination diets fail to remove all dietary triggers, and that is why I consider this diet plan the very best for autoimmune recovery. See my specific plan for this autoimmune diet below, but here are some other important steps I have taken:

- I take selenium, vitamin D, and zinc daily.
- I have eliminated nonfermented soy, which is found in most soy products. Soy can cause a decrease in thyroid function.
- I now take the necessary steps to avoid the stress of "drama and trauma" in my life.
- I take a probiotic supplement each day to help heal my gut.
- I make sure to get at least eight hours of sleep whenever possible.
- I don't take life so seriously anymore. Once you have cancer, you learn it does not pay, health wise, to "sweat the small stuff."
- I try to schedule a monthly massage to help release stored muscle tension.
- I take a daily walk (now that I am able to do it again!).

What to Eat to Get Back on Your Feet

Autoimmune disease cannot be cured, but it is possible to put it into remission. My diet includes no grains and no refined sugar at all, but it does include many other food items that are tremendously helpful for an ailing system.

The main and most important components of this diet are meat, seafood, and eggs. It is important that you source them, however, and try to get these foods from animals that are fed foods that are natural to them, organic, and non-GMO. Free-range chicken and beef and wild-caught fish are ideal.

The diet also includes ample amounts of vegetables and low-glycemic fruit, such as blueberries and strawberries, plus healthy fats like coconut oil and avocado. Nuts and seeds are allowed after a few weeks.

Ultimately what I have outlined here and find to be a great help in my continued recovery is the Paleo diet. Nutrient dense, the Paleo diet is whole foods–based and allows you to eat seafood, eggs, meats, seeds, fruits, and vegetables. I have found it to be very easy to implement.

The goal is to improve your health by providing your body with balanced and complete nutrition and avoiding processed, refined foods and empty calories. Like I have said for many years, "If it doesn't rot or sprout, do without."

I have adopted this way of eating, and have done so after researching and finding a plethora of evidence, both peer reviewed and anecdotal, that the diet does indeed help those with autoimmune disease not only manage their symptoms, but even begin to reverse the disease or at least halt its progression.

I have seen incredible results not only in myself but also in clients who were able to successfully put the Paleo autoimmune protocol into practice. These clients have eliminated many of their symptoms, whether they were suffering from Hashimoto's disease, Sjogren's syndrome, psoriasis, rheumatoid arthritis, multiple sclerosis, or another disease. It is amazing to see a person's health turn around after she implements a diet change, especially when the disease she is dealing with has taken so much life away from her. This is truly a case of food being medicine and medicine being food!

I find that following a Paleo diet is actually simple. I also like to refer to this way of eating as the autoimmune recovery diet.

The following foods are allowed (remember, no GMOs):

- All meat, organic and grass fed
- All seafood, wild caught
- Eggs, organic
- Vegetables, all kinds
- Fruits, all kinds
- Edible fungi, like mushrooms
- Nuts and seeds

WHY IS PALEO THE WAY TO GO?

While there are many other dietary programs out there, I personally have found that Paleo works well for me and my children. I especially like it because the foods support the basis for a thriving digestive system. Simply by including the right foods and eliminating others, you set up a great environment of health-promoting probiotics in the gut. This diet emphasizes prebiotic and probiotic foods that build powerful immunity, while at the same time it does not include the foods that contribute to leaky gut (gut dysbiosis). The integrity of gut barrier tissues is critical to your objective of building a dynamic immunity. Some foods contribute to the health of these tissues, while others tear them down. The Paleo diet includes the good ones and avoids the bad ones that are hard to digest, which irritate and damage the very tissues you need to build up. Just remember, when your gut barrier is breached (as in leaky gut), autoimmunity is certain to be reached.

I like to refer to this approach as "eating the rainbow." Just think yellow, blue, green, orange, and purple when you choose your fruits and vegetables, and enjoy them all. While you're eating all these delicious foods, you probably won't even realize how good they are for you, but your body will quickly recognize all of the health-building benefits. Who wouldn't want to improve his or her cardiovascular risk ratios, reduce inflammation, improve glucose tolerance, lose weight, and improve autoimmune issues, all without taking any drugs? All of these results have been proven in clinical trials on the Paleo diet. When I learned of the benefits of the Paleo diet, especially concerning autoimmunity, quickly implementing this way of eating was a no-brainer for me.

What sold me the most about the Paleo way of eating was the realization that it reduces dangerous inflammation and promotes proper activity of the immune system. This can change everything for you! How does it do it? Some foods encourage inflammation, and with the Paleo diet, those foods are out! Only foods that support your immune system are in! If these conditions are in play, your struggling immune system can actually recover. The really great news is that the game doesn't have to be over. You have a fighting chance, and this is where you begin when you intend to win!

The Paleo way of eating is really not a diet, but a way of life. Your focus is long-term health. I can attest that once your health is in jeopardy, you will make any change in your lifestyle or eating habits that will lead your body back to health!

Can you do it long term? Yes! Adopting a Paleo diet fully illustrates "eating to live." Many people have great gains in their health by avoiding foods that are known to spark inflammation in the body. You should learn to live without wheat, soy, peanuts, pasteurized and industrially processed dairy, and any foods that are processed using chemicals. If you don't want to ignite inflammation, don't eat any of these foods that are major triggers.

WHAT FOODS HAVE TO GO WHEN YOU GO PALEO?

The answer is easy—foods that trigger inflammation have to go.

The Paleo diet excludes the following:

- Grains and pseudograins such as amaranth, buckwheat, and quinoa
- Most legumes, with the exception of those with edible pods like green beans
- All dairy, but especially pasteurized and processed products (please note that if you are sensitive to dairy, you also may be sensitive to grain)
- Foods and sugars that are refined and processed with chemical additives and preservatives
- Refined seed oils like canola oil and safflower oil

There you have it. There are many wonderful books on the Paleo lifestyle. I can attest that it does great things for anyone who is the victim of an autoimmune attack. Since this book focuses on catching the "elusive butterfly" of thyroid disease, I want to suggest that you learn all you can about this new way of eating (which is actually a very old way of eating, in that our ancestors ate this way, and they experienced less degenerative disease and virtually no autoimmunity—at least, none that I have found in any of my research).

We are living in much different times, with triggers all around us. If we are not triggered by unrelenting stress, crime, bad news reports, or financial and family issues, it is the food that we have to choose from, much of which has been genetically altered, processed, and is full of preservatives, chemicals, and artificial colors that cannot be found in nature. Now more than ever, you must be proactive in terms of your health. As I have always said, "If it doesn't rot or sprout, do without." If you have autoimmune thyroid disease, this is imperative!

When to Test for Sensitivities

If you follow the Paleo diet/autoimmune protocol and still feel unwell, I recommend that you get tested for food sensitivities. The Paleo protocol isn't always enough to discover which foods are causing your immune system flares. If your symptoms aren't improving on a strict autoimmune prevention diet, or if you've been eating a Paleo diet and your symptoms do not abate or they start to come back, you may still be eating a food that is inciting an immune response.

This is a good case for getting a food sensitivity test to determine exactly which foods are the culprits. Typically most autoimmune thyroid patients get their testing done through Cyrex Labs, which test for both IgG and IgA antibodies and can detect intolerances to a wide variety of foods.

They have recently released a test called Array 10, which covers a great deal of foods in both cooked and raw form. This test is beneficial to a person on the Paleo diet who is not seeing the improvements they were hoping for. Array 4 is another Cyrex test frequently used for patients who are unsure whether they are intolerant to dairy, eggs, or other foods that are commonly associated with a gluten cross-reactivity response.

It is important to note that these tests are only accurate if you've eaten the food in question within the past four to six weeks. If you have been dairy free for six months, testing for a dairy sensitivity likely wouldn't give you a positive result, even if you are truly intolerant. The testing option is more suited to people who have been eating some of the questionable foods recently and have experienced a return or exacerbation of symptoms.

If you feel that you need to be tested to determine which foods might be an issue for you from an immunological standpoint, I strongly recommend working with a qualified practitioner who can help you navigate the testing options and interpret the results of your tests.

PALEO PAYS OFF

To close out this chapter on the autoimmune recovery diet, I would like to share with you the story of physical therapist Ann Wendell:

> "All of your blood work looks fine. The only thing that comes up is thyroid antibodies, but that's nothing to worry about."
>
> My primary care doctor said these words to me in 1999, after I told him I'd been feeling anxious and jittery and couldn't sleep for days at a time. I'd just had my first child a few months before, so since nothing else could be determined, the most obvious diagnosis was that I had postpartum anxiety and depression.
>
> But while the symptoms went away over time with treatment, they were soon replaced by a mind-numbing fatigue. Little did I know that my own body

was in the process of attacking itself because of an autoimmune disease called Hashimoto's thyroiditis.

Fast-forward to 2007. I had been under a tremendous amount of stress over the year. Though I continued to exercise, somehow I gained almost twenty pounds, and my hair began falling out in clumps. Even after eight hours of sleep, I was still so exhausted I could barely get out of bed in the morning.

I began researching my symptoms. My doctor's words came back to me, and I began reading everything I could find on thyroid disorders. After getting an ultrasound, I discovered I had nodules on my thyroid.

So with medication, over a few months I began to feel like I was getting some energy back. But my weight didn't change....

The impact this disease had on my life in the beginning was huge. I had been an athlete my entire life, swimming competitively in college, running 10Ks, and doing triathlons. At thirty-seven, I suddenly found myself unable to walk three miles with my children. To say that I was afraid for my future would be an understatement.

About a year into treatment for Hashimoto's, I mentioned to a coworker that I felt better but still not great. He suggested I try going gluten free for a few weeks. I resisted, because I loved cereal, bread, and pasta. But then I learned that celiac disease is an autoimmune disease, and people with one autoimmune disease are more likely to be diagnosed with others over the years. I decided to give it a go.

After two gluten-free weeks, I felt 80 percent better. I was feeling more energetic, and gone were the cramps and painful bloating. I began to lose a little bit of weight.... That was two years ago.

Then last spring I heard rumblings about the Paleo

> lifestyle. I researched the principles and learned that grains like wheat, rye, and barley can cause damage to the gut lining and put people at high risk for autoimmune diseases, including Hashimoto's thyroiditis, type 1 diabetes, and lupus. I went Paleo and cut out all of my gluten-free treats and dairy, increased my intake of coconut milk and oil, and began consuming larger quantities of grass-fed meats.
>
> Almost immediately I noticed a difference in how I felt. My joint and muscle pain slowly faded away, I felt more rested when I woke up in the morning, and my brain felt sharp again. I even lost most of the weight I had gained over the years.
>
> In the six months since I went Paleo, I've gone from not being able to walk a few miles to running, hiking, rock climbing, and weight lifting. My blood work looks good, my thyroid nodules are smaller, and I feel like I'm back to living the healthy life I had before Hashimoto's decided to wreak havoc on my body.

In Ann's story—and in my case too—it's about eating to live instead of living to eat. May you find this to be a life-affirming and life-sustaining way to live as well.

Epilogue

A DELICATE DANCE

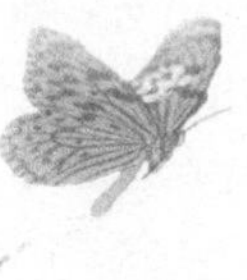

FEELING HELPLESS IS one of the most rapid ways to deplete the function of your thyroid and adrenal glands. I remember how helpless I felt when no answers were forthcoming for my daughters and me during the months and years leading up to, and even after, our diagnoses.

Once you are finally diagnosed, the next hurdle is finding a health-care provider that actually will partner with you, hear you, and treat you—*you*, not just a set of numbers on a blood work report. It can be scary and bewildering to give your power to someone else hoping that they know what they are doing just because they have a license to practice medicine and to prescribe medicine. Unfortunately many health-care providers do not know how to treat thyroid disease optimally, let alone the adrenal component. It is you who must know when to "fire your doctor" if you are not improving. You do not have the luxury of spending months or years with prescribed treatment that is not helping you get your life back.

Once you realize that you may be dealing with thyroid disease, you will have to, in essence, become your own physician. You will have to be your own advocate—or the advocate of someone you care for—and PUSH! (Remember, PUSH—Push Until Something Happens. You can do this!)

Often smoldering thyroid disease raises its ugly head

after a significant event in your life, such as an emotional trauma, divorce, illness, accident, or a recent surgery. I call these *triggers*. It may be that you experienced a string of traumas within a relatively short period of time. In other words, "when it rained, it poured," in terms of stressful life events. That was the case for me—a chain of very stressful life events over which I had no control. Finally illness had control over me.

It took years of going from one doctor to another. One specialist after another told me it was all stress. Yes, stress was part of the picture. But my thyroid and adrenal glands were underfunctioning, and not one physician considered it to be a possible cause for my fatigue, shortness of breath, sinus and bladder issues, hypoglycemia, anxiety, panic attacks, and the increasingly difficult time I had recovering from common illnesses.

If Hashimoto's Were an Onion

Hashimoto's hypothyroidism is so much more than a thyroid disease. It is a whole-body disease. If you want to feel better, you must peel away any and all triggers, much like peeling an onion. And yes, just like when peeling an onion, there are tears involved, because this illness can rob you of years of vibrant health.

Where do you start?

1. It all begins with the diagnosis. Ask your doctor to test your thyroid antibodies. If you have them, you have Hashimoto's. And if you do not have antibodies, you might still have Hashimoto's. This can be tricky, and your clinician must have a good understanding of Hashimoto's in order to identify it in this case.

2. After your diagnosis, you must eliminate all food triggers that contribute to gut inflammation and the resultant leaky gut. This especially includes gluten and all grains. Some people start by eliminating dairy and eggs as well.
3. Take a good probiotic to help repair the gut ratio (good to bad bacteria).
4. Learn to balance your blood sugar. Eat lean and green every three hours to keep your blood sugar stable. This will keep the stress off your adrenals (and you).
5. Take thyroid medication. Armour or Nature-Throid are my top choices for this. Many physicians prescribe Synthroid, but remember that Synthroid is a synthetic medication that only contains T4. While it works for many people, there is a large segment of thyroid patients who do very well on Armour or Nature-Throid since these contain T4, T3, T2, and T1, which is what our thyroid normally produces.
6. Get adrenal support. Ashwagandha, pantothenic acid, vitamin C, or adrenal glandular supplements help most people. Some people may require hydrocortisone in a physiological dose because of very low cortisol levels. Have an ASI (adrenal stress index) test to see where your cortisol level is. Without adequate cortisol, your thyroid medication will not be utilized effectively and you will not feel better.

7. Give yourself stress relief and release. Do all you can to destress your life. Stress is oftentimes the trigger that starts the autoimmune ball rolling. Heal relationships, let go, let God, and move on. Your body needs your full attention now. Learn to live in the moment, and do not dwell on your condition, no matter how bad you are feeling. I know it may be hard. I have been there.
8. Find the right doctor. You want a doctor who knows to treat the patient rather than a TSH level on a blood test. Many patients suffer because their physician treats the test and not them.
9. Give it time and patience. This is one of the hardest ones to do. If you have undiagnosed thyroid disease, you have spent plenty of time being ill, and have already had to exercise much patience as you tried time after time to find out what in the world was wrong with you. Now that you have your diagnosis, you can relax in the fact that you finally know what it is. You are not crazy, you are not a hypochondriac, and you are not dying.

GO GENTLY WITH YOURSELF—THEN FLY

As you have learned, the world is quite hard on our thyroid gland. There is no need for us to complicate it even more by not expressing our feelings or not making our voices heard. Burying our emotional needs can wind up burying us. Our food and water are full of pesticides and hormones; we are exposed to radiation from microwaves;

we fall victim to heavy metal exposure; and there is no shortage of toxins in our cleaning products, beauty products, and sunscreen. In addition, continual high stress levels and constant dieting can drain and tax the thyroid. This is our current daily culture.

The thyroid governs many functions in the body, so having a thyroid condition carries a lot of implications. Your thyroid regulates your blood sugar, body temperature, bone health, energy level, metabolism, menstrual cycle, cholesterol, heart rate, organ function, brain function, and stress hormone response. Most importantly, your thyroid regulates the quality of your life. Your thyroid plays a vital role in balancing your entire body. Is it any wonder that you feel so ill and your life feels so disrupted when this important gland malfunctions?

I now live my life without a thyroid. It is not easy, but I do all the things I have shared with you each day, and I manage to enjoy my life. I continue to speak my truth, even if my voice shakes. Eliminating triggers, changing my lifestyle, managing my intestinal health, and keeping strict with my follow-up scans have been part of my personal road to recovery from Hashimoto's and papillary thyroid cancer. Through lifestyle interventions like removing food sensitivities, changing diet, balancing the gut flora, treating infections, addressing nutrient depletions, and removing triggers, many individuals, including myself, have been able to eliminate symptoms and reduce autoimmunity, and even reverse it in some cases.

My youngest daughter and I now live life "thyroidless." While we are grateful the cancer was found, we know that there is an underlying autoimmune issue we must continue to address for the rest of our lives through diet, targeted supplements, lifestyle change, and the practice of gratitude and prayer.

In closing, here is a message to you from my daughter Jillian:

> Dr. Janet, otherwise known as Mom to me, is writing this book to talk about the struggles we have been through together fighting this battle called thyroid disease and autoimmune disease. What I can tell you is, you are not alone. You will get through this! If my mother's story and my story can help you, then this journey has been worth all the struggle. Like Mom always said, there is a reason for everything, and we believe that God is good and has a plan for us! I'm happy to say that this chapter in God's book of my life is over and now He has something great for me and my mom.

My prayer is that a person who complains of fatigue and mysterious, life-disrupting symptoms will be tested for autoimmune thyroid markers sooner rather than later, in days not decades. I also pray that people who have subclinical hypothyroidism and complain of fatigue, weight gain, hair loss, and other thyroid symptoms receive a trial of thyroid medications. My prayer continues for persons who do not feel well on T4-only medications like Synthroid, who need to be given an opportunity to try combination T3 and T4 medications, like Armour or Nature-Throid.

Most importantly I hope that the medical community will dust off and fine-tune their listening skills when it comes to their patients who come to them with this "invisible illness" called thyroid disease, and better yet, any autoimmunity. Finding the cause is better than any drug, surgery, radiation, or chemo. It is better than simply masking the symptoms.

In the meantime I encourage you to take charge of your health. Learn as much as you can about thyroid disease, about Hashimoto's, and about autoimmunity, and demand better care. Remember to PUSH.

My goal is to free you from your cocoon of unwellness. I hope this book has been wind beneath your wings. You deserve to fly!

With many blessings,
Dr. Janet

NOTES

Introduction—You and Your Undiagnosed Thyroid Disease

1. Byron J. Richards, "New Insights on Thyroid Function and Human Intelligence," Wellness Resources, January 25, 2013, accessed October 10, 2015, http://www.wellnessresources.com/health/articles/new_insights_on_thyroid_function_and_human_intelligence/.
2. "General Information/Press Room," American Thyroid Association, accessed October 10, 2015, http://www.thyroid.org/media-main/about-hypothyroidism/.
3. Ibid.; Mary Shomon, "Top Ten Signs That You May Have a Thyroid Problem," About Health, accessed October 10, 2015, http://thyroid.about.com/cs/basics_starthere/a/10signs.htm.
4. "General Information/Press Room," American Thyroid Association.
5. Ibid.
6. Ibid.
7. "About Thyroid Cancer," AACE Thyroid Awareness, accessed October 10, 2015, http://www.thyroidawareness.com/thyroid-cancer.

Chapter 1—My Story

1. Datis Kharrazian, *Why Do I Still Have Thyroid Disease Symptoms* (Carlsbad, CA: Elephant Pres, 2010), 23.

Chapter 2—Get to Know Your Thyroid

1. M. Shimakage et al., "Expression of Epstein-Barr Virus in Thyroid Carcinoma Correlates With Tumor Progression," *Human Pathology* 34, no. 11 (November 2003), http://www.ncbi.nlm.nih.gov/pubmed/14652819; K. Mori and K. Yoshida, "Viral Infection in Induction of Hashimoto's Thyroiditis: A Key Player or Just a Bystander?" *Current Opinion in Endocrinology, Diabetes and Obesity* 17, no. 5 (October 2010): 418–424, http://www.ncbi.nlm.nih.gov/pubmed/20625285.

Chapter 3—You, Your Doctor, and the Elusive Butterfly

1. "General Information/Press Room," American Thyroid Association.

2. M. N. Akcay and G. Akcay, "The Presence of Antigliadin Antibodies in Autoimmune Thyroid Disease," *Hepatogastroenterology* 50 (December 2003): Suppl. 2, cclxxix–cclxxx.

3. M. Alevizaki et al., "TSH May Not Be a Good Marker for Adequate Thyroid Hormone Replacement Therapy," *Wiener Klinische Wochenschrift* 18 (2005): 636–640.

4. All items in this list are taken from "Why the TSH Lab Test Is not Enough," ThyroidChange, accessed October 13, 2015, http://www.thyroidchange.org/about-testing.html.

5. Ibid.

6. Ibid.

7. Ibid.

8. Ibid.

9. "Well Women Guide to Scoliosis," Well-Woman.com, accessed November 30, 2015, http://www.well-women.com/scoliosis.html

10. Meredith Melnick, "Are You at Risk for Congestive Heart Failure?," *TIME*, March 23, 2011, accessed October 14, 2015, http://healthland.time.com/2011/03/23/are-you-at-risk-for-congestive-heart-failure/.

11. Ibid.

12. Ibid.

13. Elizabeth Sporkin, "As Fans Rally With Cards and Sympathy, Elizabeth Taylor Once Again Battles for Her Life," People.com, May 14, 1990, accessed October 14, 2015, http://www.people.com/people/archive/article/0%2C%2C20117645%2C00.html.

14. "Elizabeth Taylor: 'I Can't Face Any More Operations,'" *Telegraph*, accessed October 14, 2015, http://www.telegraph.co.uk/news/celebritynews/7539949/Elizabeth-Taylor-I-cant-face-any-more-operations.html.

15. Sporkin, "As Fans Rally With Cards and Sympathy, Elizabeth Taylor Once Again Battles for Her Life"; "A Partial List of Liz Taylor's Medical and Personal Maladies," FindaDeath.com, accessed October 14, 2015, http://www.findadeath.com/Deceased/t/Elizabeth_Taylor/Elizabeth_Liz_Taylor_Illnesses_maladies.htm; Sheila Marikar, "Hollywood Icon Elizabeth Taylor Dies at Seventy-Nine," ABC News, March 23, 2011, accessed November 18, 2015, http://abcnews.go.com/Entertainment/hollywood-icon-elizabeth-taylor-dies-79/story?id=12894882.

16. "Enlarged Heart: Causes," Mayo Clinic, accessed November 30, 2015, http://www.mayoclinic.org/diseases-conditions/enlarged-heart/basics/causes/con-20034346.

17. Mary Shomon, "Celebrity Thyroid Patients," AboutHealth.com, accessed October 14, 2015, http://thyroid.about.com/od/newscontroversies/ig/Celebrity-Thyroid-Patients.--02/index.htm.

18. Ibid.

19. Ibid.

20. Ibid.

21. Ibid.

22. Ibid.

23. Mike Falcon, "Rod Stewart Faces Thyroid Cancer," *USA Today*, February 22, 2011, accessed October 14, 2015, http://usatoday30.usatoday.com/news/health/spotlight/2001-02-22-stewart-thyroid.htm.

Chapter 4—Thyroid Cancer

1. "Thyroid Nodules Usually Not Cancerous, but Should Be Treated: NetWellness," The Plain Dealer, May 1, 2013, Cleveland.com, accessed October 13, 2015, http://www.cleveland.com/healthfit/index.ssf/2013/05/thyroid_nodules_usually_not_ca.html.

2. Ibid.

3. Ibid.

4. Arnold L. Goodman, "Incidence and Types of Thyroid Cancer," EndocrineWeb, accessed October 13, 2015, http://www.endocrineweb.com/guides/thyroid-cancer/incidence-types-thyroid-cancer.

5. Ibid.

6. Ibid.

7. Ibid.

Chapter 5—The Thyroid and Adrenals

1. H. D. Abdullatif and A. P. Ashraf, "Reversible Subclinical Hypothyroidism in the Presence of Adrenal Insufficiency," *Endocrine Practice* 12, no. 5 (September–October 2006): 572.

2. "What is Adrenal Fatigue?," AdrenalFatigue.org, accessed October 14, 2015, https://www.adrenalfatigue.org/what-is-adrenal-fatigue.

3. Ibid.

4. Ibid.

5. "Tests for Adrenal Fatigue You Can Do At Home," Thyroid Patient Advocacy, accessed November 18, 2015, http://tpauk.com/main/tests-for-adrenal-fatigue-you-can-do-at-home/.

6. T. Yamada et al., "An Increase in Plasma Triiodothyronine and Thyroxine After Administration of Dexamethasone to Hypothyroid Patients With Hashimoto's Thyroiditis," *Journal of Clinical Endocrinology and Metabolism* 46, no. 5 (1978): 784–790.

7. "Are You Experiencing Stress-Related Adrenal Fatigue?," AdrenalFatigue.org, accessed October 14, 2015, https://www.adrenalfatigue.org/.

CHAPTER 6—THE THYROID AND THE HEART

1. Irwin Klein and Sara Danzi, "Cardiovascular Involvement in General Medical Conditions," *Circulation* 116 (2007): 1725–1735.

2. "How Thyroid Hormones Impact Your Heart," Thyroid Federation International, accessed October 15, 2015, http://thyroidweek.org/en/thyroid-and-heart/how-thyroid-hormones-impact-your-heart/.

3. "Cardiovascular Disease in Women," World Heart Federation, accessed October 15, 2015, http://www.world-heart-federation.org/press/fact-sheets/cardiovascular-disease-in-women/.

4. "Merck Serono Supports Seventh International Thyroid Awareness Week to Unmask Hypothyroidism," Merck KGaA, accessed October 15, 2015, http://www.emdgroup.com/emd/media/extNewsDetail.html?newsId=67D7B46D75F2E476C1257E4E005514EC&newsType=1.

5. Mayo Clinic Staff, "Hyperthyroidism (Overactive Thyroid)," MayoClinic.org, accessed November 18, 2015, http://www.mayoclinic.org/diseases-conditions/hyperthyroidism/basics/complications/con-20020986.

6. N. Caraccio, E. Ferrannini, and F. Monzani, "Lipoprotein Profile in Subclinical Hypothyroidism: Response to Levothyroxine Replacement, a Randomized Placebo-Controlled Study," *Journal of Clinical Endocrinology & Metabolism* 87, no. 4 (2002):1533–1538.

7. Ibid.

8. A. E. Hak et al., "Subclinical Hypothyroidism Is an Independent Risk Factor for Atherosclerosis and Myocardial Infarction in Elderly Women: the Rotterdam Study," *Annals of Internal Medicine* 132, no. 4 (February 15, 2000): 270–8.

9. B. Müller et al., "Impaired Action of Thyroid Hormone Associated with Smoking in Women with Hypothyroidism," *The New England Journal of Medicine* 333, no. 15 (1995): 964–9.

10. Caraccio, Ferrannini, and Monzani, "Lipoprotein Profile in Subclinical Hypothyroidism."

Chapter 7—The Thyroid and Blood Sugar

1. "General Information/Press Room," American Thyroid Association.

2. Ibid.

3. Chris Kresser, "Thyroid, Blood Sugar, and Metabolic Syndrome," July 23, 2010, accessed October 16, 2015, http://chriskresser.com/thyroid-blood-sugar-metabolic-syndrome/.

4. Ibid.

5. Ibid.

6. David Mendosa, "Hypothyroidism and Diabetes," Health Central, January 26, 2011, accessed November 19, 2015, http://www.healthcentral.com/diabetes/c/17/130112/hypothyroidism/

7. Merella Hage, Mira Zantout, and Sami Azar, "Thyroid Disorders and Diabetes Mellitus," *Journal of Thyroid Research* 2011 (2011), Article ID 439463, http://www.hindawi.com/journals/jtr/2011/439463/.

8. S. Lenzen, H. G. Joost, and A. Hasselblatt, "Thyroid Function and Insulin Secretion From the Perfused Pancreas in the Rat," Endocrinology 99, no. 1 (July 1976):125–129; L. Gullo et al., "Influence of the Thyroid on Exocrine Pancreatic Function," Gastroenterology 100, no. 5, pt. 1 (May 1991):1392–1396.

Chapter 8—The Thyroid and Autoimmunity

1. Kharrazian, *Why Do I Still Have Thyroid Disease Symptoms.*

2. "General Information/Press Room," American Thyroid Association.

3. Justin Marchegiani, "Hashimotos and the Gluten Connection," *Celiac Handbook*, July 25, 2014, accessed November 18, 2015, http://celiachandbook.com/hashimotos-and-the-gluten-connection/.

4. Soo-Jee Yoon et al., "The Effect of Iodine Restriction on Thyroid Function in Patients with Hypothyroidism Due to Hashimoto's Thyroiditis," Yonsei Medical Journal 44, no. 2 (2003): 227–235, http://www.eymj.org/Synapse/Data/PDFData/0069YMJ/ymj-44-227.pdf.

5. Kharrazian, *Why Do I Still Have Thyroid Disease Symptoms.*

CHAPTER 9—THE THYROID AND THE BRAIN

1. Marchegiani, "Hashimotos and the Gluten Connection."
2. Dr. Craig A. Maxwell, "Anxiety Attacks Caused by Food," Ask Dr. Maxwell, January 1, 2014, accessed November 18, 2015, http://www.askdrmaxwell.com/2014/01/anxiety-attacks-caused-by-food/.
3. Dr. Datis Kharrazian, "Got Brain Drain? Hashimoto's and Brain Degeneration," Dr. K. News, September 25, 2013, accessed November 18, 2015, http://overmeanly22.rssing.com/browser.php?indx=12108508&last=1&item=6.
4. Ibid.
5. Daniel G. Amen, "Thyroid Balance—Your Key to Brain and Body Harmony," Amen Clinics, May 20, 2014, accessed November 18, 2015, http://www.amenclinics.com/blog/thyroid-balance-your-key-to-brain-body-harmony/.
6. Ibid.
7. Dana Trentini, "Are You Living Life With Thyroid Brain Fog?" *Hypothyroid Mom* (blog), October 24, 2014, http://hypothyroidmom.com/are-you-living-life-with-thyroid-brain-fog/.

CHAPTER 10—THE THYROID AND MENOPAUSE

1. "Thyroid and Menopause: Confusing the Symptoms," WebMD, accessed November 19, 2015, http://www.webmd.com/menopause/guide/symptoms-thyroid-vs-menopause.
2. W. K. Nicholson et al., "Prevalence of Postpartum Thyroid Dysfunction: a Quantitative Review," *Thyroid* 16, no. 6 (2006): 573–82.

CHAPTER 12—THE THYROID AND THE GUT

1. William Parker, "Lack of Breastfeeding Is a Key Factor in Autoimmune and Allergy Pandemic," Best for Babes, September 4, 2012, accessed November 19, 2015, http://www.bestforbabes.org/lack-of-breastfeeding-is-a-key-factor-in-autoimmune-allergy-pandemic/.
2. Heather Kathryn Ross, "The Truth About C-Sections, Probiotics, and the Bacteria in Your Gut," April 24, 2015, accessed December 1, 2015, http://www.healthline.com/health-news/the-truth-about-c-sections-probiotics-and-the-bacteria-in-your-gut-042415#1.
3. "Fewer 'Good Gut' Bacteria in C-Section Infants," MedicalNewsToday.com, August 8, 2013, accessed December 1, 2015, http://www.medicalnewstoday.com/articles/264473.php.

Chapter 13—Against the Grain

1. Jeffery Smith, "Genetically Engineered Foods May Be Far More Harmful Than We Thought," The Westin A. Price Foundation, October 2013, accessed December 1, 2015, http://www.westonaprice.org/health-topics/genetically-engineered-foods-may-be-far-more-harmful-than-we-thought/.
2. Chris Keenan, "Top 10 Most Common GMO Foods," Cornucopia Institute, June 19, 2013, accessed November 19, 2015, http://www.cornucopia.org/2013/06/top-10-most-common-gmo-foods/.
3. "Genetically Modified Foods," American Academy of Environmental Medicine, accessed December 1, 2015, https://www.aaemonline.org/gmo.php.
4. "Genetically Modified Foods (GMO) Linked to Tumors, Allergies and Early Death," DrAxe.com, accessed December 1, 2015, http://draxe.com/genetically-modified-foods-gmo-linked-tumors-allergies-early-death/.
5. Edward Group, "What Is the Bt Toxin?" Global Healing Center, July 22, 2013, accessed December 1, 2015, http://www.globalhealingcenter.com/natural-health/what-is-the-bt-toxin/.
6. K. Fredericksen et al., "Occurrence of Natural Bacillus Thuringiensis Contaminants and Residues of Bacillus Thuringiensis-Based Insecticides on Fresh Fruits and Vegetables," *Applied and Environmental Microbiology* 72, no. 5 (May 2006): 3434–40,
7. "Monsanto: Don't Sue the State of Vermont," Sum of Us, accessed November 19, 2015, http://action.sumofus.org/a/monsanto-sues-vermonts/.
8. Ibid.
9. Anthony Samsel and Stephanie Seneff, "Glyphosate, Pathways to Modern Diseases II: CeliacSprue and Gluten Intolerance," *Interdisciplinary Toxicology* 6, no. 4 (December 2013): 159–184, http://www.ncbi.nlm.nih.gov/pmc/articles/PMC3945755/; "The Real Reason Wheat Is Toxic (It's Not the Gluten)," The Healthy Home Economist, accessed November 19, 2015, http://www.thehealthyhomeeconomist.com/real-reason-for-toxic-wheat-its-not-gluten/.
10. Ibid.
11. The Healthy Home Economist, "The Real Reason Wheat Is Toxic."
12. Samsel and Seneef, "Glyphosate, Pathways to Modern Diseases II"; The Healthy Home Economist, "The Real Reason Wheat is Toxic."

13. Samsel and Seneff, "Glyphosate, Pathways to Modern Diseases II."

14. Dana Trentini, "Gluten: Why Hypothyroidism Patients Often Fail to Get Better," August 21, 2014, accessed November 19, 2015, http://hypothyroidmom.com/gluten-why-hypothyroidism-patients-often-fail-to-get-better/.

15. "Five Unexpected Sources of Gluten That Aren't Food," Huffpost Healthy Living, September 7, 2013, accessed November 19, 2015, http://www.huffingtonpost.com/2013/09/07/non-food-gluten-products-sources_n_3791886.html; "Seven Foods You Never Knew Contained Gluten," Huffpost Healthy Living, August 19, 2013, accessed November 19, 2015, http://www.huffingtonpost.com/2013/08/19/surprising-foods-with-gluten_n_3769463.html.

RESOURCES

Organizations

American Thyroid Association
www.thyroid.org
Dedicated to scientific inquiry, clinical excellence, public service, education, and collaboration.

ThyroidChange
www.thyroidchange.org
Dedicated to improving the diagnosis and treatment of thyroid disease through a physician-patient cooperative approach.

National Academy of Hypothyroidism
www.nahypothyroidism.org
Dedicated to the promotion of scientifically sound and medically validated concepts and information pertaining to diagnosis and treatment of hypothyroidism.

The Institute for Functional Medicine
www.functionalmedicine.org
Serving the highest expression of individual health through the widespread adoption of functional medicine as the standard of care.

Books

Cordain, Loren. *The Paleo Diet: Lose Weight and Get Healthy by Eating the Foods You Were Designed to Eat.* Hoboken, NJ: John Wiley & Sons, 2011.

Institute for Functional Medicine. *Textbook of Functional Medicine.* Gig Harbor, WA: 2010.

Kharrazian, Datis. *Why Do I Still Have Thyroid Symptoms? When My Lab Tests Are Normal*. Carlsbad, CA: Elephant Press, 2010.

Myers, Amy. *The Autoimmune Solution*. New York: HaperOne, 2015.

Wilson, James. *Adrenal Fatigue: The 21st-Century Stress Syndrome*. Petaluma, CA: Smart Publications, 2001.

Wolf, Robb. *The Paleo Solution: The Original Human Diet*. Riverside, NJ: Victory Belt Publishing, 2010.

Testing and Supplements

Consult your health-care provider for Nature-Throid:

RLC Labs
www.rlclabs.com

For autoimmune testing, contact:

Cyrex Labs
www.cyrexlabs.com

Many functional medicine practitioners use Cyrex Labs. Cyrex Array #5 is a comprehensive panel looking for a multitude of autoantibodies. The results are not a diagnosis but are suggestive of current or future autoimmune conditions. Cyrex can help catch them years before what can be considered an official diagnosis. The markers include markers for the pancreas, brain, bone, thyroid, heart, liver, gut, joints, testes, and ovaries. It does not capture every antibody known to man, but it does offer a wide variety and the markers that have been found to be the most specific and the most predictive.

Identifying the pathology early can be a blessing, if you so choose. It provides an opportunity for prevention.

For an anti-gliadin antibody (gluten sensitivity or celiac) stool test, contact:

Enterolab
www.enterolab.com
Enterolab provides a home kit for antibody testing for gluten sensitivity. This is done on a stool sample sent into the lab from your home. The kit also includes a cheek swab for genetic testing.

CONNECT WITH US!

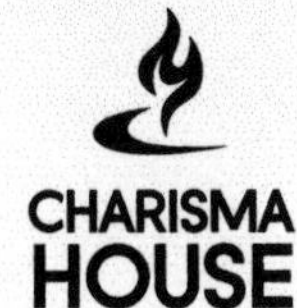

(Spiritual Growth)

Facebook.com/CharismaHouse

@CharismaHouse

Instagram.com/CharismaHouseBooks

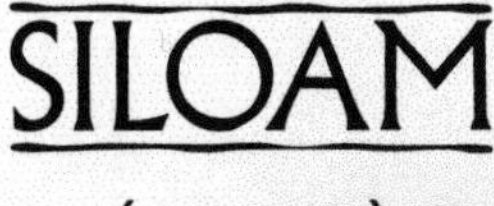

(Health)

Pinterest.com/CharismaHouse

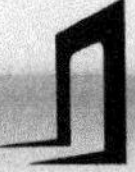

REALMS

(Fiction)

Facebook.com/RealmsFiction